USMLE®
Step 2 CS
Complex Cases

Fourth Edition

ALSO FROM KAPLAN MEDICAL

Print

Kaplan Medical USMLE® Step 2 CS Strategies, Practice & Review

Dr. Pestana's Surgery Notes

Programs

Kaplan Medical USMLE® Step 2 CS Qbank Comprehensive Courses

Kaplan Medical USMLE® Step 2 CS Practice Exam

USMLE®
Step 2 CS
Complex Cases:
Challenging Cases for Advanced Study

Fourth Edition

Edited by Felise Milan, MD

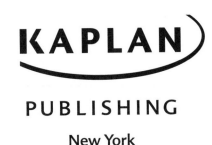

PUBLISHING

New York

© 2016, 2013, 2009, 2007 by Phillip Brottman, MD, MS

Published by Kaplan Publishing, a division of Kaplan, Inc.
750 Third Avenue
New York, NY 10017

10 9 8 7 6 5 4 3 2 1

ISBN-13: 978-1-5062-0832-9

Kaplan Publishing books are available at special quantity discounts to use for sales promotions, employee premiums, or educational purposes. For more information or to order books, please call the Simon & Schuster special sales department at 866-506-1949.

Contents

About the Writers

Felise Milan, MD, is currently a professor of Clinical Medicine at Albert Einstein College of Medicine and member of faculty in the Primary Care and Social Internal medicine residency at Montefiore Medical Center. She is the director of the Ruth L. Gottesman Clinical Skills Center and course director of the pre-clerkship clinical skills curriculum, and she directs the third-year Clinical Skills Assessment and Review Programs.

Dr. Milan received her medical degree from Albert Einstein College of Medicine and completed her residency training (in Primary Care Internal Medicine) and fellowship (in Psychosocial Medicine) at Brown University. Following her training, Dr. Milan joined the faculty at Brown to direct the psychosocial and complementary/alternative medicine curricula for internal medicine residents and the medical interviewing course for first-year medical students.

Dr. Milan's teaching and research interests include clinical skills teaching and assessment, simulation in medical education, feedback in medical education, integrative medicine, and counseling for behavior change.

Phillip Brottman, MD, MS, received his medical degree at the University of Illinois. He has fulfilled many roles, including medical director of an emergency department and member of the teaching faculty of a large community hospital with ties to a major university and a full complement of residency programs. Dr. Brottman joined the faculty of Kaplan Medical in 2004, molding the Step 2 CS curriculum and lecturing in the Step 2 CS live classes in Chicago.

For Test Changes or Late-Breaking Developments

kaptest.com/publishing

The material in this book is up to date at the time of publication. However, the Federation of State Medical Boards (FSMB) and the National Board of Medical Examiners (NBME) may have instituted changes in the test after this book was published. Be sure to carefully read the materials you receive when you register for the test. If there are any important late-breaking developments—or any changes or corrections to the Kaplan test preparation materials in this book—we will post that information online at *kaptest.com/publishing*.

Preface

The USMLE Step 2 CS exam continues to evolve, increasing the complexity and level of challenge that each patient encounter presents. This edition of *USMLE Step 2 CS Complex Cases* has been revised to match that level of complexity and to prepare the student who is ready to move beyond basic cases.

How can you best prepare for the challenges presented by Step 2 CS?

1. Make sure you are completely familiar with all the rules and procedures for the test format.
2. Develop an open-ended style of information-gathering, and let the patient fully tell their story. Don't close your focus early in the interview—keep several possible diagnoses in mind.
3. Don't go zebra hunting. USMLE wants to know that you will recognize diagnoses that present commonly and diagnoses that are dangerous to miss.
4. To the best of your ability, fully suspend disbelief as you enter each encounter: Pretend that these are real patients with real problems who need your help.

Another important way you can prepare to excel on Step 2 CS is to practice working up unfamiliar patient cases *by yourself*. A common reason that students are unsuccessful on this exam is that they have insufficient experience doing their own clinical reasoning. Students in US medical schools receive excellent training as part of a medical service or team, but clinical training rarely requires them to do their own clinical reasoning on a "fresh" case. By the time any individual student does their history and physical and starts to think about a case, many others have already done so and there is a working analysis of the patient's problems. So after their year of clinical clerkships, students often have a falsely elevated estimation of their ability to walk into a room without any prior knowledge of the patient, take a thorough history, do a focused physical exam, and create a differential diagnosis.

This book can help you change that. You can use the cases in this book interactively with friends, family, and colleagues to practice clinical reasoning when you are not influenced by what clerkship you are on or how others have conceptualized the case. Practice your time management by strictly timing your practice encounters (15 minutes) and note writing (10 minutes). Ask your "patients" to give you honest and constructive feedback on what it was like to be your patient: Did they feel listened to and respected? Did they feel you were empathic and engendered their trust?

No single study tool can cover all possible clinical problems that might be presented in Step 2 CS, but this book provides significant breadth and depth. Mastery of the cases in this edition will get you well on your way to passing the exam and ready for internship.

Best of luck!

Felise Milan, MD
Editor

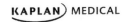

The Basics

THE PURPOSE OF THE EXAM

The USMLE states: "Step 2 of the USMLE assesses the ability of examinees to apply medical knowledge, skills, and understanding of clinical science essential for the provision of patient care under supervision, and includes emphasis on health promotion and disease prevention. Step 2 ensures that due attention is devoted to the principles of clinical sciences and basic patient-centered skills that provide the foundation for the safe and effective practice of medicine." (usmle.org)

To accomplish this, the two USMLE Step 2 exams make sure that you have the basic skills needed to function as a first-year resident. Step 2 Clinical Skills (CS) is a clinically based exam with standardized patients to test your ability to perform as a first-year resident. To that end:

- You need to look professional and act and speak like a doctor.

- USMLE has made it clear that they want you to approach these encounters as if you are at least an intern. Approach the encounters and discuss the case as if you are the responsible physician. While you can mention that you will consult with other physicians, do not assign all responsibility for decision-making to an imaginary resident or attending.

- You must be able to collect the pertinent history and perform a focused physical exam while supporting the patient's emotional and physical needs.

- You must be able to convey in writing your history and physical findings, as well as the diagnoses, diagnostic reasoning, and diagnostic tests required, to the grading physician.

WHERE TO FIND INFORMATION ABOUT THE EXAM

There is only one place to obtain accurate, definitive, and up-to-date information about all aspects of the Step 2 CS exam, and that is from the USMLE itself. While you are studying for this exam, make a habit of regularly going to www.usmle.org. Do not rely on social networking sites to get your information. It is important to get the "rules of the game" directly from those responsible for developing and grading the exam.

The USMLE Step 2 CS Content Description and General Information booklet contains detailed information about what you need to bring and what to expect the day of the exam; it can be downloaded as a PDF file. It also explains that "irregular behavior," if observed, can be noted and reported with your scores. Make sure to visit the USMLE website for any notifications or announcements.

HOW THE EXAM IS SCORED

Step 2 CS is a pass/fail exam made up of three separate subcomponents, each of which is also pass/fail. If you fail one subcomponent, you fail the entire exam and you will then need to retake the entire exam another day. All three subcomponents must be passed on the same day. The three subcomponents are:

1. Spoken English Proficiency (SEP)
2. Communication and Interpersonal Skills (CIS)
3. Integrated Clinical Encounter (ICE)

You are not graded on the basis of your passing or failing on each patient; instead, your pass/fail determination is based on your overall performance in the ICE, CIS, and SEP across all 12 cases. Even if you get off to a bad start on a case, do your best and get as many points as possible for each of the three subcomponents. Don't let a bad performance on one case follow you to the next one. Take a deep breath and head into the next case with a positive attitude. If a case seems particularly challenging or different from the other cases, it is possible that it was an unscored pilot test case.

Spoken English Proficiency (SEP)

This section is graded by the Standardized Patient (SP) on a rating scale that is most likely the same for all 12 cases. This score is graded while you are writing your Patient Note. The big question is: Can you understand the SP, and can the SP understand you? Clarity of verbal English communication is the key. Word pronunciation, word choice, and minimizing the need to repeat questions are important. However, no human communication is perfect, and USMLE does not require you to be perfect either. You will not be graded down just because of an accent.

Communication and Interpersonal Skills (CIS)

This section is also graded by the SP. Again, the checklist has been developed based on national consensus documents as to essential communication skills. It tests your bedside manner and skill in questioning the patient. Specifically, the SP is looking at your questioning skills and information-sharing skills, as well as your professional manner and rapport.

Integrated Clinical Encounter (ICE)

The ICE subcomponent tests your ability to gather and interpret data. The data gathering is the history and physical you collect. A change made in 2012 eliminated the history checklist completed by the SP. On the current exam, the only history for which you receive credit is what is documented in your note. The physical exam is evaluated by the SP based on which maneuvers were done during the encounter. The data interpretation is the diagnoses you list, and the supporting history and physical you cite as justification for your diagnoses. The tests ordered and the overall impression of the Patient Note are graded by the physician. So the physician grades the majority of the ICE component.

Standardized/Simulated Patients (SPs)

You will have taken an exam like this one before, but you may not have mastered this testing format. The Step 2 CS exam assesses interpersonal skills, cognitive skills, and complex psychomotor skills all at once. The SPs you see are trained to portray patients with certain disease states or problems. They know what to say and do depending on the actions and speech of the doctor. SPs are trained by the National Board of Medical Examiners to portray the patient case and be able to report what took place. They are trained on the physical exam criteria, so they can evaluate not only whether a physical exam maneuver was attempted but also whether it was done correctly. They do not have professional degrees in health care; in fact, many of them are actors. However, SPs certainly do know how they want to be treated by their physicians. Because the SPs grade the CIS portion of the exam, it is impossible to pass if you don't treat them as real patients all the time. For this reason, it is important that you do not speak to the SPs outside of the role of a patient.

COMMUNICATION AND INTERPERSONAL SKILLS (CIS)

The CIS component of Step 2 CS relates to fostering the relationship, gathering information, providing information, helping the patient make decisions about next steps, and supporting emotions. USMLE emphasizes that the SPs will be evaluating the student's ability to demonstrate patient-centered communication by treating the patient with respect, showing interest in the patient as a person, and showing empathy for the patient's condition. This section of the exam is just as important as SEP or ICE. Having excellent communication skills is necessary for success in the real world as well as on Board exams. The Communications and Interpersonal Skill (CIS) checklist will be the same for each of the 12 patients you see on Test Day.

Expressing Empathy

As part of your role as doctor to the SP, you will need to be empathetic. Being empathetic means being sensitive and understanding of the patient's emotional and physical state. By your actions and words, you show the patient that you understand how he feels and that you respect his concerns. You demonstrate by your actions and speech that you want to work together and help improve the patient's comfort and health. No patient wants to be dismissed as someone whose problems are not worthy of your attention.

Express empathy early in the encounter. It is much easier to win over your patient's trust early in the interview by using empathy than to do so later in the interview.

Respond to the Patient's Emotions

Pay careful attention to any emotions that are expressed, whether expressed verbally or nonverbally, and respond to them. Some key verbal cues are hearing the patient say that they are "worried," "scared," or "concerned," or using any similarly emotionally charged word.

Express Empathy Through Appropriate Touch

It is sometimes appropriate to use touch to get the patient's attention. This is especially useful when a patient is crying. Touch only the shoulder or forearm—never the leg. Do not grab, pat, squeeze, or rub the patient. Never sit on the patient's bed.

Tips for Communication with the SP: Establish Rapport

Tip 1. Communicate as you would with a real patient.

Do your best to forget this is not a real patient. Treat the SP as you would a real patient.

Tip 2. Pay attention.

Listen! This is the most common problem in communication: Doctors do not listen to their patients. While the patient is speaking, concentrate on what he or she is saying. Do not think about what your next question will be. If you have to write yourself a note on the clipboard, look down at it only briefly. Many doctors score low on all elements of the exam because they were not listening.

Tip 3. Do not interrupt the patient.

If you ask a question, let the patient answer. Do not speak again until the patient is finished speaking! Yes, this can be hard to do. The cases are designed and scripted to be doable in the 15 minutes allotted. Interrupting is seen by the patient as rude. In addition—though it may seem counterintuitive—interrupting often slows you down, because asking and answering questions takes longer than simply listening to the patient's story. However, there is one exception when it comes to not interrupting your patient: When your patient is rambling and talking about unimportant, perhaps tangential, issues. It is a challenge to you—and part of the case—to see if you can gently redirect the interview. An effective strategy is to acknowledge what they have just told you, and then refer to something else they said and ask a related question. For example, "I can see how upsetting it is when your sister talks about you behind your back. You said that Saturday was the first time you had chest pain. Can you tell me more about that episode of chest pain?"

Tip 4. Carefully observe your SP's body language.

If the patient is crying, grimacing, or displaying overt emotions or discomfort, it is part of the case! Comment on it and respond to it empathically.

Tip 5. Use facilitation skills.

Using good eye contact, saying "uh-huh," nodding your head, and repeating the patient's last word or phrase can all be effective ways to convey that you are listening and to encourage the patient to keep telling their story. Do not hide behind the clipboard. Hold it so it does not cover your face or mouth. It is normal to look down occasionally at your clipboard when you write notes. If you nod up and down slightly when writing on your clipboard, it communicates that you are still listening.

Tip 6. Keep a professional, confident demeanor.

SPs are looking to see if you are calm, confident, concerned, and caring. Both verbal and nonverbal communications are important. How you stand or sit can project calmness or nervousness. Whether standing or sitting, don't move or fidget a lot, shifting your weight back and forth. You will appear nervous if you constantly tap your pen, touch your hair, or twist your ring. Nervous physicians make for nervous patients. Patients start to wonder if the doctor really knows what he is doing when he acts nervous.

Tip 7. Be aware of your nonverbal behavior.

Facial expression is part of nonverbal communication. Generally, if the patient is in no distress or is smiling, you should be smiling as well. If the patient is in distress, is in pain, has respiratory distress, or is crying, you should drop the smile and look calm, caring, and confident. You do this by pretending this is a real-life patient whom you want to help. Your facial muscles will then take care of themselves.

Your tone of voice is also important. Never be angry or condescending or appear uncomfortable when you ask delicate questions. Practice the parts of the History several times until you can ask the Sexual History with the same ease as the History of Present Illness (HPI).

Be especially careful not to cross your arms, as this projects disapproval to the patient.

Tip 8. Be nonjudgmental.

One of the ethical tenets of being a physician is to be nonjudgmental. Even if we personally disapprove or find patients' habits undesirable, we are not to reveal our personal feelings. We treat and care for everyone with the same respect. Speech is the easiest thing to control, but it's important to keep your facial expression, body language, and tone of voice from showing any disapproval as well.

If the patient feels he is not being judged, he'll be more receptive to counseling. In the context of counseling, there is no conflict between counseling and being nonjudgmental. We are expected to help patients change behaviors that can be damaging to their health. The key is that we are basing our recommendations on medical science and, we hope, are offering realistic advice our patients can comply with.

Tips for Communication with the SP: Gathering the History

Tip 1. Summarize and clarify all unclear information.

If you aren't sure what the patient has said, you could ask the question in another way. The most important thing here is to paraphrase and find out what the patient is trying to convey. Summarizing back to the patient what you think he said can be a very effective way to clarify information, confirm you've been listening, and lead you to your next question.

Tip 2. Use open- and closed-ended questions.

You will need to use a combination of open- and closed-ended questions. Open-ended questions allow the patient to tell his story in his own words. This is often the quickest way to obtain the history. In general, start by asking open-ended questions, and use closed-ended questions to fill in the gaps of information you need to collect. When you move on to a new topic, repeat the pattern. With the elimination of the history checklist completed by the SP, the SP is now much more free to answer your open-ended questions with valuable information.

Tip 3. Try not to ask leading questions.

A leading question is a closed-ended question that presumes the physician knows the answer and is just checking. Leading questions are often judgmental and encourage the patient to say what he thinks the doctor wants to hear, even if it isn't the truth. For example:

> *Leading question:* "You work, don't you?"
> *Nonleading question:* "Do you work?"

If you do not assume or presuppose the answer to a question, you can avoid this pitfall.

Tip 4. Ask only one question at a time.

You will find that you can ask questions fairly quickly and wait for the patient's response. If you ask several questions at once to save time, however, you end up wasting time trying to get the patient's true meaning. Typically, if you ask more than one question, the SP will answer only the last question asked.

Tip 5. Use transitional statements.

Transitional statements inform the patient of what is coming next in the encounter. At a minimum, use transition statements before the family history, the sexual history and other areas of social history (to reassure about confidentiality), and closing transitions. Keep the statements short. All you need to say is what is going to happen next; you are not explaining the reason why. Finally, do not use transitions in the form of a question. You are not asking permission from the patient; you are merely telling her what to expect next. Here are examples of the most common times in the patient encounter when you will need to make a transitional statement.

Before the Past Medical History (PMH)

> **Doctor:** "Now I'm going to ask you about your health in the past."

Before the Family History (FH)

Inform the patient that you are no longer talking about her but now want to know about her family.

Before Starting the Sexual and Social Histories

Inform the patient about confidentiality. If you do not do this, the patient may not provide all the information you need. Typically, confidentiality needs to be stated just once. Occasionally you will meet patients who will not give you the HPI until you assure them your conversation is confidential.

Before the Closing

> **Doctor:** "Let me tell you what I am thinking."

Tips for Communication with the SP: Providing Information

Tip 1. Use lay language when speaking with patients; avoid medical jargon.

Avoid medical terminology. Speak to patients as much as possible with lay terminology. Patients are often shy or intimidated by a doctor's technical and highly educated speech.

In addition, it is inadvisable to give long, technical explanations. Just use the lay terms to describe medical tests and procedures. If you use medical jargon, the SP will pretend not to understand. You can use a technical term only if the patient uses it first. Even if the SP is portraying a physician who is a patient, do not use medical jargon.

Almost every physician makes an occasional mistake by using medical terminology with a patient. If you get caught by your SP or you realize you have made a mistake, you can correct yourself:

> **Doctor:** "I'm going to ask for a CBC—that is, a blood test to look for infection and anemia."

Tip 2. Avoid the pitfalls of being reassuring.

Patients like physicians who are reassuring. The problem is, it is tempting to promise that you can cure the patient. But no workup or test results are available, and the diagnosis is not yet fixed, so no definite prognosis can be made at this time. Also, many patients are sophisticated enough to realize they have just been made a promise that cannot be kept.

You're better off reassuring the patient that you:

- Understand his concerns.
- Will do everything you can to make him feel better.
- Will do everything you can to find out what is wrong.
- Will get him the best treatment available.
- Will remain his doctor and will always be available to help.

The Introduction

The introduction can be thought of as four tasks:

1. Entering the room
2. Greeting the patient
3. Offering a handshake
4. Asking the first question

Task 1. Entering the Room

At the beginning of the case, you will be standing outside the door with your clipboard. You will hear the overhead announcement, "Your patient encounter will now begin." Do not write on your clipboard until you hear the starting announcement.

Read the Doorway Information carefully and take up to 45 seconds to collect your thoughts about the case. We recommend writing the patient's name as it appears on the doorway across the top in large letters. If you forget the patient's name while in the room, you can glance at this as a reminder.

Next, write the vital signs under the name. That way they will be ready to transcribe onto the Physical Exam section of the Patient Note. Some doctors like to write out a schema or template to guide their history-taking. Some doctors also like to write out the differential diagnoses before entering the room.

When you are ready to enter the patient's room, knock twice loudly on the door. Take a deep breath, let it out, smile, and enter. There is no need for you to wait for the patient to respond verbally before you enter.

When you enter the room, notice whether the patient is in street clothes. This will reinforce whether the case will involve history and possibly counseling but no physical exam.

Task 2. Greeting the Patient

Say hello, and tell the patient your name and your role. Always use the appropriate title (Mr., Mrs., Ms.) unless the patient specifically gives you permission to use the first name.

Task 3. Offering a Handshake

The handshake is a traditional greeting. Handshaking is the generally accepted convention, regardless of the gender or age of the patient or of the doctor. Deciding on whether to shake hands or not can be simplified into three general rules.

Rule 1. Always shake hands if the patient offers. It would be considered rude to refuse.

Rule 2. Do not initiate a handshake if the patient has any emotional or physical distress. You would not want to extend your hand to someone in significant pain or with a possible injury. If the vital signs are abnormal, consider whether the patient is in distress. Similarly, a patient in emotional distress will typically not appreciate the contact. Looking at the patient's face will help you decide if a handshake is helpful or not.

Rule 3. When in doubt, leave it out. You may occasionally meet a patient from a cultural background where you may not be sure about the handshake. If you aren't sure, it's better to err on the safe side and leave it out.

If you decide to shake hands, offer your hand when you say "Hello."

Task 4. Asking the First Question

The first question must always be an open-ended question, such as:

> **Doctor:** "How can I help you today?"

This is an excellent way to begin the interview. It shows that you are caring and want to help. Here are three of many alternative ways to begin:

> **Doctor:** "What brings you in today?"

or

> **Doctor:** "What can I do for you today?"

or

> **Doctor:** "I see you have *(state the symptom listed on the doorway)*. Please tell me all about it."

The key here is to be sure it is an open-ended question. Do not begin the interview by making small talk or commenting about the weather.

After you ask your opening question, be quiet, listen, and let the patient tell you their story.

The Closing or Summary

The summary is completed after you finish your physical exam. A complete closing consists of seven tasks:

1. Making the transition
2. Summarizing what you've heard
3. Giving knowledge
4. Telling what you think needs to happen next/Negotiating what happens next
5. Counseling as needed
6. Asking for questions
7. Saying goodbye

Task 1. Making the Transition

This is to let the patient know that you have finished your physical exam and now want to tell him what you think: "Let me tell you what I am thinking."

Task 2. Summarizing What You've Heard

The purpose of this is to highlight the key historical points and the key physical findings. It is your last chance to make sure you have the information correct. There is no need and no time to repeat everything the patient told you.

Task 3. Giving Knowledge

This is where you explain in lay language and without medical jargon what you think might explain the patient's symptom(s) or problem(s). It is perfectly acceptable to be unsure of the exact diagnosis. After all, you have not even done any tests yet or—in cases that might need a breast, pelvic, or rectal exam—done a full physical exam.

Task 4. Telling What You Think Needs to Happen Next/Negotiating What Happens Next

In this section, be definite. While you're yet unsure of the final diagnosis, you can be certain about what tests you think need to be ordered. Depending on the nature of the test, there might be some negotiating involved. For example, if you think that a cardiac catheterization is needed, this might involve some negotiating with the patient to agree to an invasive test.

Task 5. Counseling

If you have found any behaviors that affect a patient's health, this is the time to advise the patient on the importance of treatment. Counseling about smoking, alcohol abuse, drug abuse, addiction of any kind, safe sex practices, depression, domestic violence, weight loss, and management of chronic diseases such as hypertension and diabetes would all be appropriate here. For any of these issues, it is key to first figure out the patient's stage of readiness to change the behavior. If you haven't already, find out what are the patient's reasons for continuing the behavior and what might be the obstacles to changing it. Simply telling the patient that they need to change the behavior is not usually a successful strategy.

Task 6. Asking for Questions

You want to ask the patient at least once if they have any questions. Give them time to formulate their question, and send signals that you really want to hear their questions. A quickly asked, perfunctory request for questions that is rapidly followed by another statement or question will send the message that your request was not sincere.

The patient may ask you a very challenging question that has the potential to make you defensive, uncomfortable, or unsure of how to answer. Try to find out what concern underlies their question and how you can best address it, and ALWAYS express empathy for the patient's concern.

Task 7. Saying Goodbye

This is the last step in the closing. It is a nice touch to end by telling the patient that you are glad they came to see you today, or something similar and appropriate to the context. If applicable, you can thank them for all the information they provided and give a last reassurance that you will do everything in your power to help them.

What Should You Do If You Run Out of Time? At the end of the 15 minutes with the patient, you will hear the announcement "This encounter is now over." As soon as this announcement is made, you stop earning points. You will not get credit for any additional history you obtain, physical you do, or counseling you give.

Even worse, the clock is now running on the 10 minutes that remain for you to write your Note. So you need to get out of the room—fast. The SP also wants you to make a rapid exit. The SP has to grade you, set up the exam room, and get ready for the next doctor. If your exit takes too long, a proctor will come into the patient room to ask you to leave.

HISTORY-TAKING

General Approach to the Content

The history you need to take on your Step 2 CS exam is different from what you did in medical school. In medical school and most clerkships, the emphasis is on completeness, especially when admitting a patient to the hospital. For Step 2 CS, you will take a focused history, gathering information relevant to the chief complaint(s) or problems(s). However, that relevant information may be things that are often relegated to the social or family history. For example, in a patient with polyuria, polydipsia, and weight loss, a family history of diabetes is indeed relevant. For a patient with asthma, smoking history is part of the HPI. In other words, you are going to skip aspects of the history that are not important in making a diagnosis, ordering tests, and counseling the patient.

Furthermore, no two histories will be the same. Sometimes the family and social histories are not important. There are even situations where there is very little history of present illness to obtain. Asking nonrelevant history is not penalized, though you could have been spending your time asking relevant questions. Your time is best spent asking questions that will help you test your hypotheses regarding differential diagnoses. As you practice, you will see that you need an organized approach and a general idea about what is relevant in different situations.

Remember, the only history content you get credit for is that which is documented in your note.

The History of the Present Illness (HPI)

To fully explore the chief complaint, consider the following aspects, which should apply to most complaints. If the case does not have a site of pain (such as chest pain or sore throat) but does have a symptom (such as fatigue, fever, or shortness of breath), have the patient begin talking about the problem. For example: "Please tell me about your symptoms."

Location

Be specific; have the patient point to the exact location. This is especially important when different structures or organs are located near each other (e.g., head/neck, abdomen).

Intensity/Quantity

The pain scale (0–10) is used only for pain; it is not used for symptoms. To determine the intensity of a symptom, ask how bad the symptom is, or ask the patient to compare it to previous symptoms. Alternatively, ask how the symptom is affecting the patient's life: What the patient can't do when pain or a symptom is present is a very valuable measure of severity. For some symptoms, such as vomiting or diarrhea, frequency or quantity is the best measure of severity.

If a patient appears to be in distress, be sure to document that finding in your physical exam as well as under general appearance.

Quality of the Symptom

Have the patient use as many descriptive adjectives as needed. If the patient does not provide useful descriptive terms, you can suggest some terms and ask them to choose. For instance: "Would you say the pain is sharp, dull, squeezing, pounding—do any of those words describe it?" If bodily fluids are involved, ask the patient to describe the fluid's consistency and color, and the presence or absence of blood.

Onset of Symptoms and Course

Knowing the onset of any pain or symptom is very important in determining possible causes of the symptom. Key questions to assess onset include:

"When did it begin?"
"What were you doing when it started?"
"Did it come on slowly? Suddenly?"

For patients who are not sure when a chronic symptom began, ask "When were you last completely well?" Onset also includes the duration and frequency. The most important aspect of course is whether the symptom is getting better or worse over time.

Radiation

Patterns of pain radiation can be helpful in determining likely diagnoses. (See the table "Typical Patterns of Pain Radiation" later in this section for more on this topic.) Do not use the term *radiation* in your questions to patients. Instead, ask the patient if the pain "moves" or "travels."

Aggravating Factors

To ascertain aggravating factors, ask the patient "Does anything make it worse?" Aggravating factors are expected for most histories. You will need to ask this question of almost all patients in the exam. (See the table "Factors That Aggravate and Alleviate Symptoms" later in this section for more on this topic.)

Alleviating Factors

"Does anything make it better?" should be asked of all patients. You may also ask the patient directly about activities that you suspect would make her symptoms better or worse.

Associated Symptoms

Associated manifestations are symptoms that a patient might have based on the diagnosis you have made. If you do not have a diagnosis in mind yet, you can ask good associated-symptom questions based on the chief complaint and the preceding history alone. Negative findings are just as important as positive findings.

For example, if you suspect that a patient with chest pain has acute myocardial infarction, you should also ask about palpitations, syncope, shortness of breath, diaphoresis, nausea, and vomiting. For any gastrointestinal symptom, you will want to ask about abdominal pain, nausea, vomiting, constipation/diarrhea, and fever. In joint-pain cases, ask about rash and fever—this may be a tipoff that you're dealing with a rheumatology case.

Previous Episodes of Chief Complaint

"Have you ever had this before?" is a question you will want to ask of all patients about any symptom. Often patients will not volunteer information from many years ago. If they don't volunteer it, ask for it specifically. For instance, if a patient has multiple episodes of recurrent headache, the diagnosis is more likely to be primary headache (e.g., migraine). If it's a new-onset headache in an older adult who doesn't typically have headaches, then consider other diagnoses such as temporal arteritis, tumor, hydrocephalus, or any hemorrhage.

Typical Patterns of Pain Radiation

Type of Pain	Typically Radiates To
Ischemic chest pain	Arms, neck, back, jaw
Kidney stone	Groin and testicle
Gallbladder	The tip of the right scapula
Spleen injury	Top of the shoulders (diaphragm irritation)
Testicular torsion	Lower abdomen
Abdominal aortic aneurysm	Back
Pancreatitis	Back
Posterior penetrating gastric ulcer	Back
Sciatica	Down leg to foot
Pharyngitis pain	Can radiate to ear

Factors That Aggravate and Alleviate Symptoms

Common Aggravating Factors	Common Alleviating Factors
Ischemic heart disease: exertion, walking up stairs, sexual intercourse	Angina pectoris: rest
Asthma: physical exertion, exposure to cold air, dust, smoking, animals	Pericarditis: sitting forward
Ulcer: eating food, taking aspirin or ibuprofen (NSAIDs)	Ulcer–GERD: antacids or eating food
Meningitis: movement, jumping up and down	Meningitis: lying down, dark room
Migraine: exposure to sound or light	Migraine: dark, quiet room; caffeine ingestion
Tension headache: stress	Tension headache: massage
Gallbladder: eating fatty foods	Gastric outlet obstruction: vomiting
Pancreatitis/gastritis: alcohol ingestion	Renal colic: moving about
Polymyalgia rheumatica: inactivity (gel phenomenon: stiff, sore joints after resting for a few hours)	Muscle spasms: heat, hot bath
Musculoskeletal pain: moving about	Musculoskeletal pain: keeping still, not moving

Past Medical History (PMH)

The PMH can be divided into four components:

1. **Major illness.** Ask the patient if they have a history of any major illnesses. In adult patients, ask specifically about certain common diseases: diabetes, high blood pressure, high cholesterol.

2. **Hospitalizations.** Ask if the patient has ever been hospitalized or stayed overnight in the hospital. You need just a one- or two-word description of why the patient was hospitalized. If a hospitalization, surgery, or procedure was recent (i.e., within the last month), consider the possibility that the current case is a complication or progression of disease.

3. **Trauma.** Ask if the patient has ever had any major injuries.

4. **Surgical history.** Ask if the patient has ever had any operations. Occasionally during the physical exam you will find a surgical scar you did not expect. If you collect the information during the physical, just remember to include it in your note.

Medications

Medication history is essential to all patient histories. By finding out what medications a patient takes every day, the physician can get a good idea of what chronic illnesses the patient has. In addition to the prescription medication(s), the physician needs to know all other drugs the patient is taking. The three medication categories are:

1. Prescription
2. Over-the-counter (OTC)
3. Vitamins and herbs

For most cases you don't need the dose, frequency, or route. You need only the name of the drug. Use whatever name the patient gives you; the trade name or generic name is acceptable.

If you are not familiar with a particular medication, ask the patient why he is taking it. Many medications are prescribed for multiple indications, so be sure to ask why the patient is taking the medication in this case too. For example, if a patient tells you that she is taking bupropion, you will need to ask if she is taking it for depression or smoking cessation.

Checking compliance is important in many patient cases, because noncompliance, medication complications, and/or drug interactions may account for some or all of the patient's symptoms—for example, the chronic congestive heart failure patient who stops taking his medicine and now is short of breath; a patient on phenytoin who takes OTC cimetidine for heartburn and presents with dizziness, slurred speech, and ataxia; or a patient with a dry cough who was recently started on an ACE inhibitor.

Common Medications and Their Side Effects

Nonsteroidal Anti-inflammatory Drugs (NSAIDs)

Common names   Ibuprofen, naproxen, meloxicam, diclofenac

Adverse reactions   Gastrointestinal (GI) bleeding, ulcer, allergic reaction, renal insufficiency

Diuretics

Common names   Furosemide, HCTZ (hydrochlorothiazide), spironolactone

Adverse reactions   Hypokalemia, hypotension, electrolyte disorder, syncope. Gout can be caused by thiazide diuretics.

Digoxin

Common names   Digoxin/lanoxin

Adverse reactions   Heart block headache, dizziness, fatigue, nausea/vomiting

Beta Blockers

Common names   Atenolol, metoprolol, naldol (anything that ends in "-ol")

Adverse reactions   Bradycardia, erectile dysfunction, hypotension, wheezing

ACE Inhibitors/Angiotensin Receptor Blockers (ARBs)

Common names   Lisinopril, enalapril, captopril, losartan, irbesartan

Adverse reactions   Hyperkalemia, cough, angioedema

SSRIs

Common names   Citalopram, escitalopram, fluoxetine, paroxetine, sertraline

Adverse reactions   Sexual dysfunction (anorgasmia), serotonin syndrome (confusion, fever, anxiety, hyperreflexia, tremors, insomnia, tachycardia, hypertension)

Statins

Common names   Atorvastatin, simvastatin, rosuvastatin

Adverse reactions   Rhabdomyolysis—muscle pain, renal failure

Patients also commonly take herbal medications to self-treat conditions. It may be useful to know a few common preparations and why patients might take them. Of course, to be sure, you should ask the patient why he is taking it.

- Saw palmetto: benign prostatic hypertrophy
- Cranberry: urinary tract infection
- Echinacea: upper respiratory infection
- Ginseng: stress and memory issues
- St. John's wort: depression

Allergies

Medication allergies are the most important information to get in most cases, especially in the case of infection, where the patient might need to be treated with an antibiotic. Antibiotic allergies are the most common of the medication allergies. If the case involves an allergic reaction—a rash, shortness of breath, runny nose, watery eyes, anaphylaxis, bee sting—a more detailed allergy history is indicated. The four types of allergens to ask about are medications, foods, animals, and plants or other environmental sources. When the presenting complaint is related to allergies, record the allergy information in the HPI.

Review of Systems (ROS)

You will not have time in 15 minutes to take a full review of systems, nor is it necessary. It is the time to see if there are other major problems that you have not yet uncovered. You can ask about any organ system that you feel is relevant, but focusing on the constitutional ROS will likely get you the most important information and give you great hints as to what might be going on.

Ask about the following in the constitutional ROS:

1. Fevers
2. Night sweats
3. Chills
4. Weight loss
5. Weight gain
6. Change in appetite
7. Fatigue
8. Sleep

When you come across history relevant to the HPI in the process of doing the ROS, remember to document it in the HPI.

Family History

The family history is relevant only if the diagnosis you are considering has a genetic or familial component. Do not ask the family history if it isn't relevant. As with other parts of the history, start with an open-ended question, "Does anyone in your family have any serious illness?" Then ask as many of the following examples as are appropriate:

"Does anyone in your family have what you have?"
"Does anyone in your family have high blood sugar, high blood pressure, or heart disease?"

Obstetrical and Gynecological History

You should ask about last menstrual period (LMP) with all women past the age of menarche; however, only women with complaints of abdominal pain, abnormal vaginal bleeding, dysuria, discharge, and morning nausea will require a more detailed Ob/Gyn history.

Obstetrical History

How to determine a patient's gravida/para/abortus (GPA) status:

G = Number of times pregnant; ask "How many times have you been pregnant?"
P = Number of live births; ask "How many times have you given birth?"
A = Number of miscarriages and abortions; ask "Have you had any miscarriages or abortions?"

For example, G2P1 describes a woman who is pregnant now and has had one live birth. G3P2A1 describes a woman who is not pregnant now and has had two live births and one miscarriage or abortion.

Gynecological History

Components of a comprehensive gynecological history are the following: LMP and characteristics of menses (regularity, cramps/dysmenorrhea, flow, cycle length, spotting and age of menarche/age of menarche), last Pap smear, vaginal discharge, and birth control.

Sexual History

The sexual history or parts of the sexual history are needed only if they are relevant to the case, especially if you think the patient could have a sexually transmitted disease. Also, ask yourself if sexual function could be compromised by the diagnoses you are considering. Examples of this are angina precipitated by sexual intercourse and erectile dysfunction caused by depression, diabetes, or beta blockers. The key is not to suddenly become nervous when asking these questions. Practice them over and over until you can ask them without embarrassment. Natural transitions, such as moving from gynecological history into sexual history, can assist with making you more comfortable with the topic. Another strategy is to ask about important relationships in social history and go from there to sexual activity. During the sexual history, it is essential to avoid making the heterosexual assumption.

Standard sexual history questions are the following:

"Are you sexually active?"
"Are your partners men, women, or both?"
"Do you use contraception? "*(applicable for those having heterosexual sex)*
"Do you practice safe sex?" *(applicable for everyone)*
"How many sexual partners have you had in the last six months?"
"Have you ever been tested for HIV?"
"Have you ever had a sexually transmitted disease?"
"Do you have any concerns about sexual function?"

Social History

Depending on the case, ask about parts or all of the social history. Taking a complete social history consists of asking about the following:

- Tobacco
- Alcohol
- Recreational drugs
- Diet/exercise
- Work life
- Home life

> *Do not use the terms "miscarriage" and "abortion" interchangeably when talking with patients. To the lay public, a miscarriage is a spontaneous abortion, and an abortion is an elective termination of the pregnancy.*

Tobacco

For smokers, assess quantity (expressed in pack-years) and dependence (patient's ability to go a long time without smoking or presence of cravings). If the HPI contains any pulmonary component, a thorough smoking history is essential and should be reported in the HPI. If the chief complaint were that the patient wants to receive smoking cessation help, you would need to know all the details of when he started to smoke, what he has tried to do in the past to stop, and what methods of quitting have and have not been successful for him.

Alcohol

Use the CAGE questionnaire

- Have you ever felt you should **C**ut down on your drinking?
- Have people **A**nnoyed you by criticizing your drinking?
- Have you ever felt bad or **G**uilty about your drinking?
- Have you had a drink first thing in the morning to steady your nerves or get rid of a hangover? (**E**ye-opener)

A positive response to any of the CAGE questions or binge drinking suggests there may be an alcohol problem, and counseling should be advised. If you have already determined the patient meets the definition of binge drinking, there is no need to ask the CAGE questions. You already know there is a problem and can go directly to alcohol counseling. (*Ewing JA. "Detecting Alcoholism: The CAGE Questionaire," JAMA 252: 1905–1907, 1984.*)

Recreational Drug Use

If the patient uses recreational drugs, find out the specific names, what route is used (ingested, smoked, snorted, or IV), and when the drug was last used. Many patients also need to be asked whether they are willing to quit, and you should find out what methods of quitting they have tried in the past.

If you don't understand the street name of a recreational drug, it is fine to ask the patient.

Common names for recreational drugs:	
Alcohol:	Booze, brews, brewskis
Amphetamines:	Speed, crank, crystal meth
Cannabis:	Hash, hashish, dope, pot, reefer, bud, ganja, weed, grass
Cocaine:	Blow, coke, toot, nose candy, crack
Benzodiazepines or barbiturates:	Downers
Heroin:	Horse, brown sugar, smack
Phencyclidine:	PCP, angel dust
Anabolic steroids:	'Roids

Diet/Exercise

Patients may not need to be asked about diet or exercise habits when presenting with acute complaints. However, if the problem relates to heart disease, diabetes, hypertension, or cardiovascular disease, diet and exercise might be relevant.

A good place to start is to simply find out how much, if any, exercise the patient gets on a regular basis. For diet, a good place to start is to find out how often the patient eats in restaurants or buys take-out food. If they cook, how often do they fry their food? Ask the patient if they drink regular soda and if they eat a lot of snack food.

Work Life

There are situations where the kind of work the patient does may give you clues about the diagnosis. A coal miner who is short of breath, for instance, may have pneumoconiosis. Also, the patient's level of stress is important. Note that the stress level is *what the patient reports,* not how stressful you determine the job to be.

Home Life

There are things you will need to know about the patient's home life:

- Who does the patient live with?
- Is there any stress at home?
- Is the patient having conflict with significant others? With other family members?
- For some patients, mostly female, it might be important to determine whether they feel safe at home if there is any indication of domestic abuse.

PEDIATRIC AND ADOLESCENT HISTORIES

Pediatric History

The younger the child, the more important the pediatric history. Once the child is an adolescent, the pediatric history is less relevant than the adolescent questions. A good way to organize your thoughts is to complete the usual introduction. Find out the name of the patient, the name of person you are speaking with, and the relationship between the family members.

Pediatric history consists of six subparts:

1. Prenatal—health of the mother during pregnancy, prenatal care, smoking or drinking during pregnancy, history of preeclampsia.
2. Birth—at full term, vaginal versus cesarean delivery, complications of labor, weight of baby.
3. Neonatal—length of hospital stay after delivery, medical problems, or problems with breathing, feeding, bowel movements, or infections.
4. Feeding—breast versus bottle fed, eating solid foods (depending on age), taking vitamins, allergies.
5. Development—normal patterns of growth, gaining weight; for babies, developmental milestones like smiling, speaking, walking.
6. Routine care—immunizations up-to-date, regular check-ups.

Adolescent History

The typical adolescent case will hinge on the main problems of an adolescent. The cases you will most likely see will mimic real-life problems and will center on issues such as self-esteem, eating disorders, sexual behavior, and/or drug use.

The mnemonic used to remember the components of the adolescent history is HEADSS: home life, education, activities, drugs, sex, and suicide/depression. If you ask a little about each category, you have covered a lot of potential problems.

- **Home life:** Who lives at home? Does the patient feel safe? Any evidence of verbal, physical, or sexual abuse?

- **Education:** Is the patient academically and socially engaged? Do they take an interest in and enjoy school?

- **Activities and friends:** Does the teen take part in extracurricular activities and social life?

- **Drugs:** Ask the patient about smoking cigarettes, drinking alcohol, and taking recreational drugs. It's often useful to ask if the teen's friends do any of these things, then lead into their own involvement.

- **Sexual identity and sexual behavior:** This is an important time to ask if the teen has figured out if they are straight, gay, bisexual, etc. It is always important to ask about safe sex and ask if the teen has a trusted source of information about sex.

- **Suicide/depression:** Ask about mood, interest in activities, and socializing. If depressed mood, any suicidal thoughts?

PHYSICAL EXAM

An Overview

HEENT	CHEST	NEURO
Inspection	Inspection	Mental status
Palpation	Palpation/respiratory excursion	Cranial nerves
Eyes	Tactile fremitus	Motor
Ears	Percussion	Sensory
Nose	Auscultation (sitting or lying)	Reflexes
Throat		Cerebellar
Lymph glands	**CARDIOVASCULAR**	
Thyroid	**Sitting**	**JOINTS**
	Carotid	Inspection
ABDOMEN	Auscultation	Palpation
Inspection	Peripheral pulses, edema, clubbing	Range of motion
Auscultation		Motor
Percussion	**Lying Back, Head Elevated 30 Degrees**	Reflect
Palpation	Jugular venous pressure (JVP)	Sensory
–Light and deep	Point of maximum impulse (PMI)	Vascular
–Rebound tenderness	Auscultate a second time	

Choosing the Physical Exam Maneuvers to Include for Each Case

The physical exam for the USMLE Step 2 CS is very focused on the patient's presenting complaint. This means simply that you should not do a complete head-to-toe physical exam like you were trained to do in medical school. For most cases, you will have 4 to 5 minutes to complete the exam. No two physical exams of your 12 patients will be the same.

For the USMLE Step 2 CS, you can divide the physical into six systems.

1. HEENT (head, eyes, ears, nose, and throat)
2. Chest
3. Cardiovascular
4. Abdominal
5. Neurological
6. Musculoskeletal (back, joints, and extremities)

Your goal is to perform physical exam maneuvers that are most likely on the SP's Physical Exam Checklist. Do the most relevant organ system first. For example, if the chief complaint is abdominal pain, you'll start with the abdominal exam. If the chief complaint is headache, start with the HEENT and neurological exams. Generally speaking, you want to perform a complete or near-complete exam on the most relevant organ systems for your case.

After completing your exam of the most important organ systems, go on to the secondary organ systems. You generally don't have to do all of the physical exam maneuvers on the less important secondary organ systems for that case. You do not need to do a heart, lung, and abdominal exam on all patients if the findings will not help you decide on the relative likelihood of the diagnoses in your differential.

Properly Examine the SP

Even though you are going to perform a brief and focused examination, it's important to do each step as you would for a real patient. This means actually listening to the heart and lungs for a few seconds. It's possible for some SPs to have crackles or wheezes. Try to appreciate in 3 seconds whether the patient has normal or hyperactive bowel sounds.

Actually do the reflexes, motor strength testing, sensory exam, and HEENT exam. Inspect, auscultate, percuss, and palpate! Do these maneuvers with the techniques you were taught in your physical exam course. Although you may have observed some incorrect techniques or shortcuts in the clinical setting, do not model those behaviors on this exam, as you will not get credit. For example, never do any part of the physical exam over the gown or drape. Always pull the leg support up so the patient's legs aren't hanging down when they are supine.

Handwashing

Before you touch the patient for a physical exam, it is mandatory that you wash your hands. You do not need to wash your hands prior to giving the drape or shaking hands during the introduction.

You may use either soap and water or hand sanitizer. Use the foot pedal beneath the sink to turn the water on so you don't need to touch the sink after you've washed your hands. Whatever you do, do not pretend to clean your hands.

Do not touch your own face after you wash your hands. If you sneeze or rub your nose, re-wash your hands before proceeding to touch the patient again.

Wearing gloves is not a substitution for washing hands. You should put on gloves after washing hands only if you have an open wound or infectious disease on your hands. Of course, if you are planning to touch the patient's saliva or any mucous membranes, you should wear gloves to protect yourself.

The Patient Gown and Appropriate Draping

Over the last few years, the USMLE has changed where the drape will be when you enter the exam room. If the drape is not already on the patient's lap when you come in, unfold it and spread it out on their lap so you don't forget to do so when you move on to the physical exam.

The SP will be wearing a patient gown that ties in the back, as well as undergarments. It is your job to keep the patient covered as much as possible; uncover only the part of the torso you need to examine. Then replace the gown to protect the patient's modesty.

The abdomen and chest should not be exposed simultaneously. To examine the abdomen, you or the patient must raise the gown. Raise it up to an inch or so above the costal margin and do your exam. Replace the gown when you are finished with the abdominal exam.

To examine the chest, you must lower the gown to an inch or so below the costal margin. This is for both male and female SPs. The gown must be replaced and retied when the chest exam is finished.

You or the patient can lower and raise the gown, depending on the circumstances. Let the patient know what is going to happen next.

Offer to remove the gown when it would be difficult or painful for the patient to do so herself. Perhaps she has a broken clavicle or is in respiratory distress. If the patient is in no distress, it is fine for her to lower her own gown.

Remember to retie the string ties on the back of the gown as soon as the gown is replaced.

Getting the patient undressed is the only time in the exam that you ask for permission. You would also need permission to remove shoes and socks. This is a common CS exam challenge—you won't find a diabetic foot ulcer (simulated physical finding) unless you look.

If the patient refuses to cooperate, explain the importance of the physical in order to determine the cause of her condition.

Physical Exam Maneuvers You Are Never Allowed to Do

You are never permitted to do the following on the Step 2 CS exam:

- Female breast exam
- Internal pelvic exam
- Rectal exam
- Genital or genitourinary exams, including inguinal hernia exam
- Corneal reflex exam

This list of forbidden maneuvers is part of the Doorway Information on each case for you to review. You also will never test the gag reflex, test the sense of smell, or swab for a throat culture.

A general guideline is that parts of the body covered with underwear are off-limits. If an SP has his underwear pulled up above the umbilicus and you need to examine his RLQ, you could ask him to lower his underwear slightly to the top of the iliac crests so you can do an exam.

Moreover, *do not hurt your SP.* The SP is subject to multiple exams every day. It is helpful for you to realize what is most uncomfortable for the patient.

Some other points to remember:

- Otoscopy might be the most potentially dangerous maneuver you are asked to perform. The key here is to not scratch the ear canal and give the patient a bloody ear. When you place the speculum into the external auditory canal, make sure not to insert it so deeply that the tip of the speculum touches the skin.

- When examining the pharynx, use a clean tongue blade and place it only one-third to one-half of the way back on the visible portion of the tongue. This way you will not gag your SP but will still be able to inspect the pharynx.

- Be sure to keep your fingernails off the patient's skin.

- Be sure your hands are dry after you wash them before touching the patient.

- Use a gentle touch, especially when palpating the abdomen. You need to be gentle, but firm and definitive. If you are too gentle or hesitant, that can indicate lack of confidence and competence.

- When checking for costovertebral angle (CVA) tenderness, do not "punch" your patient. A simple tap will do.

Simulated Versus Real Physical Findings

This is probably the hardest concept on the exam, as many of the patients don't actually have the disease they are portraying. The SPs are skillfully acting.

Accept All Physical Findings

Accept all actual physical findings on patients as real, with the exception of the vital signs. SPs are sometimes hired specifically to portray different diseases. The Board will hire some SPs who actually have physical findings, perhaps someone who has arthritis, old surgical scars, Bell's palsy, atrial fibrillation, or thenar muscle wasting from carpal tunnel syndrome. Certainly this is not a complete list.

The vital signs are the heart rate, temperature, blood pressure, and respiratory rate. Always use the vital signs from the Doorway Information when writing your note. Even if you take the SP's blood pressure yourself, write in your Note the blood pressure listed on the doorway. When considering the differential diagnosis and diagnostic workup, think only about the doorway vital signs.

Many patients will have simulated physical findings. Accept all simulated physical findings as real. An example of this is a SP pretending to have an acute abdomen. When you palpate the abdomen, the SP will grimace and possibly complain of pain. It may seem very realistic as if the SP actually has tenderness. Do not think that the patient is exaggerating or feigning illness; it is highly unlikely your cases will involve malingering.

It is easy for an SP to simulate weakness, abnormal reflex or sensory exam, and gait, among other things, but some physical findings are harder to simulate. While it is almost impossible for USME to hire SPs with severely abnormal findings on heart and lung exams, do not assume there will be no findings. There could be heart murmurs or some fixed abnormal lung sounds.

Notice All Aspects of the SP's Presentation

Smell your patients. They may smell of beer if they are supposed to be intoxicated, or fruity if they are portraying diabetic ketoacidosis. Pay attention to their behavior. If the patient is doing something unusual when you enter, that is part of the case. The SPs are not making up things as they go along—they are following a script.

Inspect the Skin Carefully

Inspection is important! Inspect the skin and comment on any simulated physical findings that need clarification. Patients may actually appear sweaty by spraying on water before you enter the room. You may see discolorations or marks on the skin that may relate to the patient's condition:

> *White powder*: Pallor, anemia
> *Yellow powder*: Jaundice
> *Purple*: Ecchymoses, bleeding disorder, trauma
> *Red*: Infection, inflammation

Don't Worry about Missing Subtle Physical Findings

It will be very difficult to test you on certain physical findings because they are transient, are faint, or require better equipment to appreciate. The physical findings you will be expected to see generally will not be subtle. Hearing a 1/6 diastolic murmur is not on the Physical Exam Checklist, whereas completing heart auscultation in four different locations on the chest wall will be on the Physical Exam Checklist for certain cases.

Another source of anxiety is ophthalmoscopy. Relax. As long as you are using the ophthalmoscope correctly, you will be fine. You may not see much, aside from the red reflex. Without a dilated pupil and a dark room, it is unrealistic to expect a detailed exam. Simply write down whatever you do see of the retina.

Position the Patient

You may examine the patient from either side of the bed. Try to minimize the number of times a patient has to sit up, lie back, and stand, as having the patient move is time-consuming. It is better, however, to move the patient multiple times than to skip vital physical exam maneuvers that will be on the SP's Physical Exam Checklist.

Communicate with the Patient during the Physical Exam

Tell the patient briefly what you are going to do next as you go through the physical exam. Do not give the patient the results of your findings now (unless, of course, the patient asks). If you think of more historical questions, you can certainly intersperse them with your exam.

Use new tongue blades, ear speculums, and cotton balls on each patient. Throw away your garbage. Try not to put the tuning fork and reflex hammer in your pocket—it is very easy to leave the patient's room with them. Also, always keep your stethoscope on your body. This way you will always leave the patient's room with it in your possession.

Once you have left the room, you will not be allowed to return. So if you left your stethoscope behind, a proctor will need to retrieve it for you.

You have already completed your focused physical exam and have the patient's vital signs from the Doorway Information. A common question is: When should the doctor take the SP's HR and BP during the exam? Since you are not going to use the results you obtain, the answer is: very infrequently. Certainly, if an SP asked you to check the BP, you would comply. Also, do take the blood pressure (BP) on any case where the patient is coming in for a blood pressure check. If the patient presents with a complaint that might indicate dynamic changes in vital signs, such as palpitations or dizziness on standing, you will likely want to recheck the heart rate or check orthostatics. Otherwise, you don't need to repeat the vital signs.

A copy of the patient's Doorway Information is also included inside the examination room for your reference.

By the time you formally begin the physical exam, some of the exam may have already been completed. You already know the vital signs, you have an impression of the patient's general appearance (GA), and you have noted any unusual patient behavior. You may already have noted obvious visible skin findings and any other physical findings. You may also have completed the mental status and psychiatric exams. Remember to write in your note all of these physical exam findings that you identified—you have completed some of the physical exam before you wash your hands.

COMPLETE PHYSICAL EXAM BY ORGAN SYSTEM

The most important and challenging part of the physical exam on USMLE Step 2 CS is to know what to include in a focused examination. You will have a limited amount of time. Each maneuver should relate to determining the likely and possible cause(s) of the patient's symptoms, or to evaluating the patient's condition.

Abdominal Exam

Do a complete abdominal exam when the chief complaint includes:

- Abdominal pain
- Vomiting
- Diarrhea

- Jaundice
- Urinary tract problem
- Pelvic pain

When you percuss and palpate, look at the patient's face. He will grimace to simulate abdominal pain.

Aspects of an Abdominal Exam

- Inspection: Look for actual scars, hernias, or makeup.
- Auscultation: Listen for 3 seconds in each of the four quadrants.
- Percussion: Two taps each on four quadrants; tap out liver size if you are seeing a jaundice case, liver case, or CHF case.
- Palpation: Palpate all four quadrants and the epigastric area for 3 seconds each. In a patient with abdominal pain, palpate the location of pain last.

Special Tests

Perform these as needed, such as Murphy's sign for cholecystitis, CVA tenderness for kidney, and maneuvers to evaluate for peritonitis or appendicitis.

Murphy's sign: Do this if you suspect cholecystitis. Place your hand gently under the right costal margin and ask the patient to take a deep breath. Positive Murphy's sign means the patient has pain with deep breathing or their breathing halts abruptly due to pain while you are pressing down.

Costovertebral angle (CVA) tenderness: Do this only if you suspect kidney stones, pyelonephritis, or other kidney pathology. You may perform this with the patient sitting, standing, lying supine, or lying on his side. Positive CVA tenderness means the patient complains of pain with a light tap.

Tests for peritonitis: Check for peritonitis only if there is abdominal tenderness on palpation; there is no need to do these maneuvers if the abdomen is nontender on palpation. When you are checking for peritonitis, you are looking to see if moderate motion or pressure on the abdomen produces pain.

- *Percuss for tenderness.* Lightly percuss over the 4 quadrants. If there is pain to light percussion, you don't need to do any other tests for peritonitis. However, you must verbally confirm with the patient that they had pain with percussion.

- *Rebound tenderness.* "Positive rebound" means the patient has more pain when you let go suddenly compared to when you push down slowly. Rebound is positive whether you press in the area of pain or in a different quadrant. There is not agreement whether rebound should be done in the area of pain.

- *Heel strike.* Strike the plantar surface of the heel in the caudal direction. If the patient reports pain in the abdomen, this is a positive sign for peritonitis.

- *Bed shake.* Shake the bed. If the patient confirms that this reproduces the abdominal pain, it is a positive test for peritonitis.

Tests for appendicitis: Do these only when you suspect appendicitis (RLQ pain) as part of your differential diagnosis.

Rovsing's sign: Positive Rovsing's is pain in the right lower quadrant with palpation of the left lower quadrant.

Obturator sign: Positive obturator sign means pain in the right lower quadrant with flexion of the hip to 90 degrees and rotation of hip.

Psoas sign: Positive psoas sign means pain in the RLQ with flexion of the right hip against resistance.

Chest Exam

Do a complete chest exam when the chief complaint includes:

- Cough
- Shortness of breath
- Chest pain
- Respiratory tract infection
- Sputum production

Aspects of a Lung Exam

Inspection: Check the patient's hands for clubbing, cyanosis.

Respiratory excursion: To do this test, stand behind the patient with the back of the patient's gown open. Tell the patient before you touch him, "I am going to push on your ribs." Then place both hands on either side of the lateral chest wall and say, "Now take a deep breath." Remember to say thank you after he complies.

Palpation: Check for chest wall tenderness.

Tactile fremitus: Place both hands on the patient's back at three different levels to compare left and right and feel for transmission of vibrations when the patient says "99."

Percussion: Tap at least two times on each side at a minimum of three different levels.

Auscultation: Listen on each side at a minimum of three different levels on the back, two levels on the front just above the nipple line. Listen for crackles, rhonchi, wheeze, or rub (listen from side to side). Listen to the back at the base of the lungs, bilaterally. Listen to the left and then the right. Next, move up and medially just below the scapula. Listen on the left and then the right. Finally, move up to about T3 dermatome level and listen between the spine and the scapula on both sides.

Common Pitfalls in the Pulmonary Exam

Pitfall	Solution
Examining through clothing	Stethoscope should be placed directly to skin, not on underwear.
Placement of stethoscope	Don't examine over scapulae.
Not comparing sides	Be sure to examine and compare right side to left side at each dermatome level.
Not listening to a full breath	Listen to complete respiratory cycle on each side.
Distractions	Do not talk when you auscultate!

Cardiovascular Exam

Do a complete cardiovascular exam when the chief complaint includes:

- Symptoms to suggest a myocardial infarction
- Chest pain
- Shortness of breath
- Pedal edema
- Syncope
- Palpitations

Aspects of a Heart Exam

A complete heart exam includes two exams: one with the patient sitting up and one with the patient supine (lying back) at 30 degrees.

The Sitting Cardiac Exam

Auscultation of neck bruit: Ask the patient to hold their breath, and listen over the carotid with the bell of the stethoscope. Listen for no more than 3 seconds.

Palpation of the carotid arteries: Note: Never palpate both carotid pulses simultaneously. You may complete this aspect of the exam in the lying-back position or sitting up.

Pulses: Do radial, dorsalis pedis, and post tibial, side-to-side or simultaneously. Check for atrial fibrillation (irregularly irregular pulse). There is no need to check brachial pulse if patient has strong radial pulse. Likewise, there is no need to check post tibial or popliteal if there is a strong dorsalis pedis.

Extremities: Press gently but firmly when checking for pedal edema. Check fingers for cyanosis, capillary refill, and clubbing.

Auscultation of the heart: Press the stethoscope to the skin, 3 seconds for each cardiac area. Listen to as near the aortic, pulmonic, tricuspid, and mitral areas as possible.

With female patients, ask the patient to lift her breast if the breast is preventing auscultation of the mitral area. Do not be concerned if you are not listening in exactly the correct location. Be sure not to place the stethoscope over the clothes or underneath the clothes.

The Supine Cardiac Exam

The exam table should be at a 30-degree incline.

Jugular venous distention (JVD): Ask the patient to look to the left and let them know what you are looking at.

Hepatojugular reflux: Do this if your patient has possible congestive heart failure.

Palpation of carotid arteries: You may do the carotid exam now instead of in the sitting position.

Point of maximum impulse (PMI): Place a flat hand or flat surface of several fingers on the chest.

Repeat auscultation: Listen again to all four areas.

Additional heart sounds: You can turn the patient on his left side to listen for S3, S4 or to palpate PMI if it cannot be felt from the supine position (consider this in a CHF case).

Neurological Exam

Do a complete neurological exam when the chief complaint includes:

- Headache
- Dizziness
- Balance or vision problem
- Numbness or tingling
- Psychiatric problem
- Memory problem
- Muscle weakness

Aspects of a Neurological Exam

- Mental status
- Cranial nerves
- Motor
- Sensory
- Reflexes
- Cerebellar
- Gait
- Specific tests

Aspects of a Mental Status Exam

There are five parts to a mental status exam:

- Orientation
- Memory
- Attention and concentration
- Language
- Obeys commands

It's best to complete all five parts of a mental status exam in patients with psychiatric disease, dementia, or altered mental status. You may limit the mental status exam to the Orientation only when you are not sure about the patient's mental status.

Phrasing for the Mental Status Exam

Orientation (to person, place, and time):

"Could you please tell me your full name?"
"What kind of place are we in?"
"What is today's date?"

Memory: Ask the patient to repeat three words after you. Let them know you will be asking them to remember these words again in 5 minutes. Record how many words out of three the patient remembers correctly.

Attention and concentration: Ask the patient to spell the word *w-o-r-l-d* backward.

Language: Ask the patient to name objects you point out, such as a pen or watch. Alternatively, ask her to repeat the phrase "No ifs, ands, or buts."

Obeys commands: Ask the patient to close her eyes. Be sure to have the patient open her eyes again after she completes your request.

The Cranial Nerve Exam

Cranial nerve 2: Use the Snellen eye chart to test vision. If the patient cannot see the eye chart, try holding up fingers to count. If that fails, see if the patient has light perception. Test peripheral vision by traditional confrontation.

Cranial nerves 2, 3: Check that pupils are equal, round, and reactive to light and accommodation (PERRLA). Check for direct and consensual reaction.

Cranial nerves 3, 4, 6 (extraocular movements): Let patients continue wearing their contacts or eyeglasses when checking visual activity. Say, "Please hold your head still and follow my finger with your eyes." For 3rd-nerve palsy, there is ptosis, a large pupil, and the eye is turned out. For 4th-nerve palsy, the patient can't look downward and inward. For 6th-nerve palsy, the eye is turned in.

Cranial nerve 5: For motor, ask the patient to clench their teeth. Place your hands on the jaw and feel the muscle contract. For sensory, use the cotton balls to test light touch. To test all three branches of the 5th nerve, touch the patient's face lightly and ask if it feels the same on both sides.

Cranial nerve 7: Ask the patient to show their teeth, smile, and lift their eyebrows.

Cranial nerves 9, 10, 12: Ask the patient to stick out their tongue and say "Ah." Check the palate for symmetrical movement (9th and 10th nerves). Check to see if the tongue goes out straight (12th nerve).

Cranial nerve 11: Ask the patient to shrug their shoulders.

The Motor Exam

A general screening motor exam is good for finding gross abnormalities in a stroke patient.

In some cases you may only need to check the muscle strength in the upper extremities. In other cases, just check the lower extremities.

The Motor Exam

Action	What It's Testing	Possible Phrasing
Pull arms in *Flexion of forearm*	C5, C6	"Now I'll check your arm strength. Do this *(demonstrate the action)* and don't let me push out."
Push arms out *Extension of forearm*	radial nerve	"Do this *(demonstrate the action)* and push hard."
Push wrists up *Wrist extension*	radial nerve	"Put your wrist like this *(demonstrate the action)*. Don't let me push down."
Place two fingers in patient's palm and have them squeeze your fingers.	median	"Squeeze my fingers."
Keep fingers together *Finger adduction*	ulnar nerve	"Put your fingers together like this *(demonstrate the action)* and don't let me pull them apart."
Keep fingers apart *Finger abduction*	ulnar nerve	"Spread your fingers apart and don't let me push them together."
Knee kick out *Knee extension*	L3-L4	"Next, I'll test your leg muscles. Please kick out."
Knee bend *Knee flexion*	S1	"Using your strength, can you pull back your legs?"
Foot bend up *Ankle dorsiflexion*	L5	"Point your foot back and hold it like that, using your strength."
Foot bend down *Foot plantarflexion*	S1	"Step on the gas, hard."
Lift knee *Hip flexion*	L2-L3	"Pick your knee up." *(while seated, dangling feet)*
Lower knee *Hip extension*	L4-L5	"Push your leg back down."

Aspects of a Sensory Exam

It is important to do the sensory exam if the patient is complaining of numbness or tingling, or has a history of diabetics.

- Check distal sensation for any orthopedic injury. Start distal and work proximal.
- When checking for diabetic neuropathy, if you have checked distal sensation and it is intact, you do not need to check proximal sensation.

Upper Extremity
- Tip of thumb (C6 dermatome)
- Tip of middle finger (C7 dermatome and median nerve)
- Tip of fifth finger (C8 dermatome and ulnar nerve)
- Dorsum of web space of hand (radial nerve)

Lower Extremity
- Just above patella (L4 dermatome)
- Lateral lower leg (L5 dermatome)
- Lateral foot (S1 dermatome)

Pain sensation (use the cotton swabs or toothpicks in the room): If using cotton swabs (sharp/dull), break the stick of a new cotton swab in half. Demonstrate by touching the patient with the sharp and dull ends with their eyes open. Then ask the patient to close their eyes and tell you if they feel a sharp or dull sensation.

Do each foot, keeping each hand in one place, and work side-to-side. Move proximally if the patient can't tell the difference.

Position sense: Test position and vibration sense for diabetics or those complaining of numbness. Grasp their toe on the lateral sides and ask them to tell you with their eyes closed if you are moving the toe up or down.

For vibration sense, ask the patient to close their eyes. Ask if they feel a vibration, then ask them to tell you when they stop feeling it.

Aspects of a Reflex Exam
- Compare reflexes from side to side.
- Only a couple of reflexes are needed in thyroid, suspected stroke, or suspected spinal cord lesion.
- For a suspected thyroid case, just test the biceps reflex. If the patient is hyporeflexic in the upper extremities, she will also be hyporeflexic in the lower extremities.
- For a sciatica case, just test the Achilles and patellar reflexes.
- For a stroke case, just test the biceps and patellar reflexes.
- To test a diabetic patient for neuropathy, just test the Achilles reflex.

Reflexes
- Biceps: C5, C6
- Brachioradialis: C6 (only if you suspect C6 lesion)
- Triceps: C7 (only if you suspect C7 lesion)
- Patellar: L4
- Achilles tendon: S1

Aspects of a Cerebellar Exam
- Finger-to-nose
- Heel-to-shin

Gait

Gait can be used to check for cerebellar function and motor function. There are several different tests you can do. These include:

- **Normal gait:** Ask the patient to walk a few steps away from you, then back to you.
- **Toe walking:** Ask patient to walk on their tiptoes.
- **Heel walking:** Ask patient to walk on their heels.
- **Tandem gait:** Ask patient to walk heel to toe in as straight a line as possible.

Aspects of the Specific Neurological Exams

- **Meningitis tests:** Check for stiff neck. If you have time for only one meningitis test, this is it.
- **Brudzinski:** Bring chin to chest. Test is positive if knees and hips flex spontaneously.
- **Kernig** (you'll remember because you have to touch the knee to do test): Flex the hip and knee, and try to extend the lower leg. Test is positive if there's pain and stiffness in the leg.
- **Plantar reflex (Babinski):** When you scratch the bottom of the foot, normal response is flexion of the great toe (plantar flexion). Abnormal response is extension of the great toe and flaring of toes (extensor plantar response). This indicates an upper motor neuron lesion (in a patient older than 6 months of age).
- **Romberg's:** Good to check in balance-problems cases. Ask the patient to stand with feet together, arms at their sides, and eyes open, then closed, for a full minute. This test is considered positive if the patient loses his balance. Stand behind the patient and reassure him that you will catch him if he becomes unsteady.

HEENT Exam

Do a complete HEENT exam when the chief complaint includes:

- Headache
- Eye pain
- Vision change
- Ear pain
- Dizziness
- Hearing loss
- Pharyngitis
- Nasal congestion
- Dysphagia/choking

Aspects of a HEENT Exam

- Inspection: For scars, abnormalities, deformities, and skin changes.
- Palpation: For tenderness and deformities of head, face, and sinuses. Check the temporomandibular joint (TMJ) if relevant. Palpate over maxillary and frontal sinuses.
- Examine lymph glands: Submental, submandibular, anterior and posterior cervical chain, pre- and postauricular, supraclavicular.

- Examine the thyroid gland. You can use an anterior or posterior approach when checking the thyroid. Ask the patient to swallow while you are pressing lightly over the thyroid. Offer them water to swallow if they have trouble.
- Test visual acuity using Snellen eye chart, first with both eyes, and then while covering each eye.

Otoscope and Ophthalmoscope

The tympanic membranes can be checked only with the otoscope, and funduscopy can be done only with the ophthalmoscope. Either tool can be used as a penlight to check pupils, pharynx, and nares.

Using the Ophthalmoscope

- *Check the eyes:* Look at the pupil, direct and consensual light response; note any abnormalities. Look twice at each eye, once for direct and once for consensual.
- *Inspect the sclera:* Look for redness or jaundice.
- *Inspect the conjunctiva:* Look for pallor or discharge.
- *Funduscopy:* Dim the lights (if possible). "Please look at this spot." Approach the patient from the side. Hold the ophthalmoscope in your right hand, hold it up to your right eye, and look in your patient's right eye. Then do the same for the left side. Hold the ophthalmoscope in your left hand up to your left eye, and look at the patient's left eye. Look for papilledema, cupping, AV nicking, and hemorrhages. In most cases you will just see the red reflex.

Using the Otoscope

- *Check the throat and oral cavity:* Look at the tongue. This allows for examination of the 9th, 10th, and 12th cranial nerves and the pharynx at the same time. If you are unable to see the posterior pharynx with the patient saying "Ahhh," use a tongue blade.
- *Examine the nose:* Push the nose up gently and look inside from a distance. Palpate the outside of the nose as needed.
- *Examine the ears:* Examine in patients with ear problems such as pain, discharge, or hearing loss. Put on a new clean ear speculum for each patient.
  - *Exterior:* Inspect the pinna, palpate over the mastoid process, and wiggle the pinna for tenderness.
  - *Interior:* Place the earpiece just on the inside of the tragus, and do not insert it deeply. When you are finished, throw out the earpiece.

Cranial Nerve 8

Check the patient's hearing for cases of ear complaints.

Weber and Rinne Tests for Hearing Loss

Do the Rinne and Weber tests only if there is hearing loss on history or physical examination.

- *Rinne:* Put the tuning fork behind the patient's ear and ask them if they can hear it. Move the fork to in front of ear and ask if they can hear it better or less well.
- *Weber:* Put the tuning fork on top of the patient's head and ask them if the sound they hear is the same or different in both ears.

**Use of a Tuning Fork to Determine the Cause of Hearing Loss:
Sensorineural Hearing versus Conductive**

Diagnosis	Hearing	Rinne	Weber
Normal	Normal	AC > BC	Equal
Conductive loss	Decreased	BC > AC	Louder on the side with the hearing loss
Sensorineural loss	Decreased	AC > BC	Louder on the normal side, softer on the side with the hearing loss

Notes: AC = air conduction; BC = bone conduction

Examining Joints

Aspects of a General Joint Exam
- Inspection
- Palpation
- Range of motion (ROM): With active ROM, the patient moves the joint on his own. With passive ROM, the patient relaxes completely and you move the joint. Do passive ROM only if there is pain or limited mobility with active ROM. Passive ROM helps determine whether you're dealing with a problem inside the joint (intra-articular) or outside the joint from the muscle or tendon moving the joint (extra-articular). If the pain and limited mobility is the same on passive and active ROM, the problem is intra-articular. If the pain is less and range of motion better on passive ROM, the problem is extra-articular.
- Motor strength and sensation

Aspects of a Back Exam
- Inspection
- Palpation: Palpate along the bony prominences of the cervical, thoracic, lumbar, and sacral spine. Do not touch the patient's underwear.
- Range of motion: Flex, extend, lateral flexion to left and right. Rotate left and right.
- Straight leg raise: With the patient supine, lift the leg (knee extended), stretching the nerve roots. If this causes pain radiating in a nerve root distribution (i.e., pain radiates below the knee and not merely in the back or the hamstrings), the test is positive. Compare left and right legs.
- Lower extremity motor strength (see "The Motor Exam," under Neurological Exam earlier in this section)
- Lower extremity sensation (see "The Sensory Exam," under Neurological Exam earlier in this section)
- Reflexes (patellar, Achilles)

Nerve Root Pain Distribution in the Lower Extremities
- At L4: Pain along the front of the leg; weak extension of the leg at the knee; sensory loss about the knee; loss of knee-jerk reflex

- At L5: Pain along the side of the leg; weak dorsiflexion of the foot; sensory loss in the lateral lower leg; no reflexes lost
- At S1: Pain along the back of the leg; weak plantar flexion of the foot; sensory loss along the back of the calf and the lateral aspect of the foot; loss of Achilles reflex

Knee Exam

With any paired organ, you must compare both sides. Many physicians like to examine the "normal" side first.

- Inspection: Look for any deformity, ecchymosis, or swelling. Compare to the other side.

- Palpation:
  - Check the skin for warmth.
  - Palpate the patella for fracture and ballot to check for effusion.
  - Palpate the lower femur and tibia and fibular head.
  - Palpate both menisci for tenderness.

- Range of motion

Don't forget distal motor, sensation, reflexes, and pulses.

- Check pulses: Start with posterior tibial and dorsalis pedis. If these are absent or decreased, check popliteal pulse.

- Check the distal sensation: Light touch, sharp and dull, in L4, L5, and S1 distribution

- Deep tendon reflexes (DTRs): Check patellar and Achilles DTRs

- Check joint stability:
  - Anterior cruciate ligament (ACL): Check for anterior drawer sign. Bend the knee to 90 degrees, pull the tibia anterior, and see if there is any pain or laxity. Negative is normal.
  - Posterior cruciate ligament (PCL): Check for posterior drawer sign. Bend the knee to 90 degrees, push on the tibia posteriorly, and see if there is any pain or laxity. Negative is normal.
  - Medial and lateral collateral ligaments (MCL, LCL): With the patient supine, support the thigh and knee flexed 20 degrees. Check for pain or laxity.

- McMurray meniscus test: Place the patient supine, hip flexed, knee completely flexed.
  - Laterally rotate the tibia and extend the leg. This is positive if it causes pain or snapping in the medial meniscus. This indicates a medial meniscus tear.
  - Medially rotate the tibia and extend the leg. This is positive if it causes pain or snapping in the lateral meniscus. This indicates a lateral meniscus injury.

Hip Exam

Physical Exam: The unique aspect of the hip exam is internal and external rotation, which can be helpful in distinguishing hip problems from those originating in the knee or back.

Ankle/Foot Exam

Palpation: It is very important to palpate for any tenderness. Use your fingertips and palpate the small bones of the foot. With the typical inversion injury that causes a sprained ankle, also check for associated injuries. Palpate the Achilles tendon, medial malleolus, base of the 5th metatarsal, tibia, and proximal fibula.

Range of motion of the ankle: Check plantar flexion, dorsiflexion, inversion, and eversion. Don't forget to check distal motor, sensation, and pulses.

Hand Exam

- **Inspection**

- **Palpation**

- **Range of motion and strength**

- **Distal vascular (capillary refill)**

- **Sensation**
  - Light touch, sharp, dull, and two-point discrimination
  - Ulnar nerve: fifth finger pad
  - Median nerve: third finger pad
  - Radial nerve: dorsum of hand at web space between thumb and second finger

- **Motor exam**
  - Ulnar nerve: finger adduction, finger abduction
  - Median nerve: finger flexion, thumb opposition
  - Radial nerve: wrist extension and finger extension

- **Carpal tunnel tests:** Positive will give pain/tingling over medial nerve distribution
  - Tinel sign: Tap on wrist over median nerve
  - Phalen sign: Put dorsum of hands together

Elbow Exam

- **Inspection**

- **Palpation:** Pay attention to the radial head

- **Range of motion:** Extension, flexion, supination, pronation

Shoulder Exam

- **Inspection:** Lower the gown and compare the shoulders; this is a good way to check for third-degree acromial-clavicular separation. Look for redness or deformity.

- **Palpation:** Feel for heat, crepitus, and pain. Check the entire clavicle, AC joint, humeral head, humerus, scapula, and anywhere else the patient complains of pain.

- **Range of motion (ROM):** Check active ROM. If any pain or limited ROM, then check passive ROM.

- **Strength:** Test external rotation with the hands behind head (as if combing the hair). Test internal rotation as if patient is touching his own scapula with his thumb. Check forward flexion; backward extension, adduction, and abduction.

- **Check distal function:** Check pulse, ulna, radial and median nerve, sensation, motor and reflex (see "Hand Exam" earlier in this section).

- **Palpation of bicipital groove (test for bicipital tendonitis):** Ask the patient first to sit and then to flex his arm to contract the biceps muscles. Palpate the bicipital groove to attempt to elicit pain.

- **Impingement syndrome:** Check for pain with abduction of shoulder.

- **Adson's test for thoracic outlet syndrome:** Radial pulse is less or absent when arm is abducted more than 90 degrees.

PATIENT NOTE WRITING

The Patient Note is a component of the ICE score and is the only component of the exam that is graded by a physician. The purpose is to see whether you document a history including the necessary pieces of information (remember, the SP no longer completes a history checklist) and to assess your ability to demonstrate your clinical reasoning. As long as you include a complete history and communicate your thoughts logically and clearly, you will score well. The physicians who grade the exam are not primarily concerned with grammar, punctuation, capitalization, or sentence structure. Even an occasional misspelled word—as long as it can be deciphered—is acceptable. Of course, before Test Day you should practice spelling words that are commonly misspelled, such as pneumonia, abscess, inflammation, and ischemia—or any other common medical term that gives you difficulties.

Physicians grading the Patient Note are concerned with content. The key to writing a good history and physical involves putting down on paper what you asked of the patient, what exam you did, and what you observed about the patient. This includes all pertinent negative as well as positive findings you uncover.

You may write out the history in complete sentences, although that makes it more difficult to finish on time. The key is to write phrases that clearly demonstrate how you are connecting the dots. With one- or two-word bullet points, that is often lost. The following example, in a case of a patient with chest pain, might be a good compromise:

> Patient c/o substernal chest pain
> 8/10 intensity, heavy crushing pain
> Started 1 hour ago
> Radiates to L arm
> Nothing makes it better, worse with walking
> Pain associated with SOB, diaphoresis, syncope
> Not associated with vomiting, fever

You are required to type your Note. If you type very slowly, you might want to invest some time in improving your typing speed.

It is essential that you become comfortable using the data entry form for recording your note prior to Test Day. (At the time of publication, the USMLE Step 2 CS practice note could be found at http://www.usmle.org/practice-materials/step-2-cs/patient-note-practice2.html.) Familiarize yourself with the format and practice how to move from one section to the next. Also acquaint yourself with the arrow buttons that can move your diagnosis from the first position to any other position. This saves time deleting and retyping. The keyboards at the test center will be the QWERTY type. If you are accustomed to another kind of keyboard, it would be worthwhile to get the correct keyboard to speed your data entry.

The form you will complete contains four sections: History, Physical Examination, Data Interpretation, and Diagnostic Study. For most cases you will need to write something in each section. But make sure you cover all four sections—it is not in your benefit to write a detailed History for the entire 10 minutes and leave the other three sections blank. As with the scoring for the ICE and CIS components, graders use a checklist for guidance in scoring your Note.

Use simple headings in the History to orient the physician grading your Note. The only place you will get credit for obtaining the proper history is on the Note. It is essential to record all the relevant history you obtained from the SP in the Note. As the old saying goes, "If you didn't document it, you didn't do it."

Physical Exam

When considering what to write on your Patient Note, follow this rule: If you observed it, asked it, and/or examined it, then write it down in your Note. Do not fabricate sections of the history and physical that you did not conduct. (In cases where the patient is not present—in a surrogate or phone case, perhaps—leave the Physical Exam section blank.)

Remember, a physician is grading your Note and is more concerned with communication of ideas than with format, punctuation, or spelling. There are many ways to write a Note, just as there are many ways to ask a question. This section will show you just one way to write an effective Note.

When considering which abbreviations to use, follow this rule: There are many abbreviations commonly accepted on the USMLE. (*See* Appendix A for a list.) There are other abbreviations, as well, which are frequently recognized by American attending physicians. However, when in doubt, write out the full word.

In the following paragraphs, text in **bold** is what you could write on a Note. Text in brackets is how you could describe the patient. So: **The patient is [good, bad]** means on some cases you might write **The patient is good** and on other cases **The patient is bad.** (Do not write brackets on your Note.)

When considering how to take notes, follow this rule for general headings:

VS or **Vital Signs**	**Chest** or **Lungs:** Chest
GA: General appearance	**ABD** or **Abd:** Abdomen
HEENT: Head, eyes, ears, nose, throat	**Neuro:** Neurological exam
CV: Cardiovascular	**Joints:** Joints in general

For a detailed exam of a single joint, write the name of the joint and always label it right or left. For example: **R wrist, L hand, R elbow, R shoulder, L hip, R knee, R ankle, R foot.** If the pain is in the right arm, you could use **R upper ext.** for "Right upper extremity." Be as specific as time allows.

Vital signs should be noted on every chart. Always write the vital signs that appear in the Doorway Information.

Vital Signs

"Vital Signs–WNL" or **"Vital Signs–NL."** If you are not sure if a vital sign is normal, simply write out the vital sign. You do not get a higher score for indicating a vital sign is normal or abnormal than for writing it out. You could write **"VS–NL except BP = 160/100."** Or you could just write out the vital signs that are on the doorway: **"VS 160/100, 82, 20, 37.6."**

If you think there could be confusion about the vital signs because they are abnormal, write out labels: **"VS–90/60, HR=38, RR 40,"** or **"VS: HR–100, T–102, RR–24, BP–60 systolic."**

Height and weight should be noted if relevant to the case. That would include a general physical or periodic health exam, a pre-employment physical, life insurance, or whenever you think it relevant. Since this doesn't appear on every Note, it is best to use labels such as **"WT–100 lb"** or **"Wt–100 kg."** Also, use units, as a patient can weigh 100 pounds or 100 kilograms. Height can be **"Ht–162 cm," "Height–162 cm,"** or **"Ht–5ft, 2in."**

General Appearance

This is the place to describe what you see and to comment on any unusual behavior. It's fine if you have some components of psychiatric or mental status here as well. Some examples are:

- **GA: NAD** (no acute distress)
- **GA: in [mild/moderate/severe] distress from [pain/SOB]**
- **GA: no distress, A&O × 3 (alert and oriented times three)**
- **GA: pt is pacing about the room in [pain/anger/rage]**
- **GA: dirty, torn clothes; smells of beer and body odor**
- **GA: quiet, flat affect; will not make eye contact**
- **GA: track marks on arms, multiple bruises**

Skin

There is no reason you could not describe skin on its own instead of describing it as a part of each organ system. Describe location, color, tenderness, warmth, pattern, and flat/raised as much as possible. For example:

- **Skin: multiple blue/red rash on upper and lower ext in sun-exposed areas. Warm & tender. No streaks.**

- **Skin: jaundice; or Skin: yellow powder on face**
- **Skin: [track/needle] marks on both arms**

HEENT

Writing the note for each organ system follows the same outline you memorized for the physical exam (Inspection, Palpation, etc.). There is no need to write subheadings for eyes, ears, etc.

A normal HEENT is given below:

> **HEENT: normocephalic/atraumatic, nontender. PERRLA. Fundi—red reflex intact, EOMI. TMs—no erythema, not bulging. Pharynx—no erythema or exudate. No nasal discharge. Lymph glands, thyroid not enlarged.**

If abnormalities on the HEENT are found, be as specific as possible. For example:

- **HEENT: tender, red, swollen pre-auricular node and pinna**
- **Head: deformity, tender, and bloody nose**
- **Head: tenderness of bilateral [maxillary sinus, cheek]**
- **Head: fine, thin hair. Exophthalmos [diaphoretic, sweating], large thyroid. [Tenderness, deformity, crepitus] to [nose, cheek, maxilla, jaw, zygoma, orbit, forehead].**

Further examples of HEENT note-writing:

- **PERRL:** (pupils equal, round, reactive to light)
- **PERRLA:** (the "A" stands for "and accommodation")
- **PERRLA: sclera clear, EOMI** (extraocular movement intact). **Extraocular muscles intact except [R 6th nerve palsy, R lateral gaze deficit].**
- **Visual fields intact, or R [temporal, nasal] visual field deficit**
- **Visual acuity: VA–20/20 OU** (OU = both eyes, OS = left eye, OD = right eye). **VA: 20/200 R eye, counting fingers 5 ft L eye.**
- **Visual acuity: L eye light perception only, OD–20/200. Fundi: flat** (no papilledema), **or Fundi: Not visualized, or Fundi–NL red reflex.**

Nose

Be as specific as possible:

> **No nasal discharge** and/or **good air entry B/L**, or **B/L thick yellow discharge or nasal septum [intact/perforated/with hole]**

Ears

- **Pinna nontender, no lesions. TM no erythema, not bulging.**
- **R TM red bulging, L NL.** (Right tympanic membrane is red and bulging, L tympanic membrane is normal)
- **TMs both with [perforation/holes] B/L**

Throat

- **Pharynx [clear, red, with exudates]**

Teeth

- [Dentition/Teeth], [poor/normal]

Thyroid

- Thyroid: [nontender/tender], [normal size/enlarged]. No nodules.
- Nontender, NL size, no nodules, trachea in midline; or Tender, enlarged, trachea shifted L

Lymph Gland

You may reference specifically or generally, depending on its importance to the case.

- Lymph glands: not swollen or tender
- Hard, tender supraclavicular lymph node
- Diffuse lymphadenopathy (seen with mononucleosis)

You may also list the particular glands that are swollen and tender, such as the following: [submandibular, submental, preauricular, postauricular, ant cervical, post cervical, supraclavicular, subclavicular] adenopathy.

Chest

Remember to do the complete chest exam (inspection, palpation, respiratory excursion, tactile fremitus, percussion auscultation) and document all of your findings.

A normal chest exam may be documented as follows:

- Chest appears NL, nontender, normal excursion, fremitus equal B/L. Lungs clear to auscultation and percussion.
- Chest without deformity, skin without rash or lesions. Lungs clear to auscultation and percussion bilaterally.

An abnormal chest exam may be documented as follows:

- Inspection: Increase AP diameter, or pursed-lip breathing, or chest with deformity or [ecchymoses/bruise] R flank, or thoracotomy scar
- Palpation: Tenderness on [R lat 8th rib, L CVA, lumbar spine, R costochondral margin]. Be as specific as possible about the area of tenderness.
- Respiratory excursion: Poor respiratory excursion or paradoxical chest wall excursion
- Fremitus: [increased/decreased] fremitus [R/L] [base/midlung field/apex]
- Percussion: [dull/hyperresonant] percussion [R/L] [base/midfield/apex]
- Auscultation: [decreased/absent] breath sounds [L/R]. Or you may have heard abnormal sounds: [wheeze, rhonchi, rub, rales] [L/R] [base/midlung/apex]

Cardiovascular

Think about the entire cardiovascular exam and write down the parts that you conducted.

A normal cardiovascular exam may be documented as follows:

CV- S1,S2-WNL, Regular rate & rhythm. No rub/gallops/murmur sitting and supine. No JVD. PMI not displaced. No clubbing, edema. Carotid, radial, DP, PT pulse NL & equal B/L. No carotid bruits.

Note: JVD means "jugular venous distension," and JVP means "jugular venous pressure." For the normal person, you could write **"No JVD"** or **"JVP NL."** Both notations are correct.

If abnormalities are found on the cardiovascular exam, be specific as possible.

Pulses
When documenting pulses, use the pulse grading scales as follows:

    0 = no pulse
    1 = decreased pulse
    2 = normal pulse
    3 = bounding or increased
    4 = aneurysmal dilatation

You may chart an abnormal or normal pulse in the following way:

   "[R/L] [radial/brachial/popliteal/DP/PT] pulse [absent/decreased/NL/bounding]"

Point of Maximal Impulse (PMI)
PMI: **PMI displaced.** If you felt the apex, you can describe its location.
For example: **PMI at anterior axillary line, 8th rib.**

Heart Rate and Rhythm
[RRR, irregular irregularly rhythm] (Note: An irregularly irregular heart rhythm is often atrial fibrillation.)
+ gallop rhythm (write this when you hear an S3 or S4 heart sound)
[1/6, 2/6, 3/6, 4/6] [diastolic/systolic] murmur is the basic notation for murmur. A murmur can be holosystolic, early, or late.

The grading scale for murmur is as follows:

    1/6 = faintest murmur
    2/6 = soft murmur
    3/6 = loud murmur
    4/6 = very loud murmur with palpable thrill when you check PMI
    5/6 = heard with stethoscope partly off the chest
    6/6 = heard with stethoscope off the chest

Abdomen
Think about the entire abdominal exam and write down the parts that you conducted. Remember Inspection, Auscultation, Percussion, and Palpation.

A normal abdomen exam may be documented as follows:

   ABD: soft, nondistended, BS+ all 4 quadrants, no bruits heard, tympanic all 4 quadrants, liver size–10cm. No tenderness or masses to light or deep palpation 4 quadrants.

If you did any additional abdominal tests, be sure to list them. When all additional tests are normal, they may documented as follows:

   Neg Rovsing's, psoas, obturator. No CVA pain. Neg Murphy's.

If any abnormalities are found on the abdomen exam, be as specific as possible:

- **ABD: [distended/obese/visible peristalsis].** Be sure to comment on any makeup or real changes in the skin.
- **ABD: R subcostal scar, ecchymosis periumbilical.** Bowel sounds **BS+**, or **BS+ all 4Q,** or **BS+, no bruits heard.** Everyone in this test has bowel sounds! Write something like this depending on how many quadrants you listened to.
- Percussion: It is very unlikely you will have a patient with significant ascites. However, if you do need to document this, simply write: + **shifting dullness,** or **dullness in flanks to percussion.**
- Palpation: + **tender [epigastrium/periumbilical/RUQ,RLQ,LUQ,LLQ], [+/−] rebound.** For tenderness you must describe where the patient has tenderness, and if there are any peritoneal signs. To be more thorough, describe whether deep or light palpation elicits pain.

Another example of an abnormal abdomen exam:

ABD: + tender in epigastrium to deep palpation only. No rebound. Neg Murphy's. Tender RLQ to lite touch. Positive rebound. + obturator, psoas, and Rovsing's.

Neurological

Think about the entire neurological exam and write down the parts that you performed.

A complete normal cardiovascular exam may be documented as follows:

Neuro: A&O×3. CN 2-7, 9, 10, 12 NL. Sensation intact all 4 ext. to light touch. Position sense and vibration sense NL B/L lower ext. Motor 5/5 all 4 ext. DTR 2/4 brachial, patella, B/L. Gait–WNL. No Kernig or Brudzinski. Neck supple. Straight leg raise negative B/L. Romberg negative. Babinski–downgoing toes B/L.

If abnormalities are found on the neuro exam, be as specific as possible.

Mental Status

If the patient only knows his/her name but not the place or date:

A & O × 1, or Alert and oriented to person only.

Cranial Nerves

You can interpret the physical finding or just describe it. For instance, **Pt points tongue out to L.** This is the same as writing: **L 12th nerve palsy.**

Writing: **Entire R side of face is weak, pt cannot close R eye** is the same as **R peripheral 7th CN lesion.**

Sensation

Describe where the patient is experiencing numbness.

- **[Decreased/No] light touch below knee B/L; no position sense L toe, R WNL**
- **Numbness R ulnar nerve distribution.** (You could draw a picture or write: Numb 5th digit R hand.)

Motor

Motor function is traditionally graded on a 0 to 5 scale:

0/5 = flaccid
1/5 = just a flicker of movement
2/5 = so weak that the patient cannot overcome gravity
3/5 = can overcome gravity
4/5 = somewhat weak
5/5 = normal

Some people also include 4–/5 and 4+/5 in the scale.

- **Motor: 3/5 RUE, other ext NL** describes someone with a weak R arm and the other three extremities normal.

You may also use regular language to describe the degree of weakness. For instance:

- **Motor: [Mild/Moderate/Severe] weakness RUE**
- **Motor: Pt with [dense paralysis/0/5] entire R side of body, L side WNL**

Reflexes

Reflexes are traditionally graded on a 0 to 4 scale.

0/4 = no reflex
1/4 = decreased
2/4 = normal
3/4 = somewhat hyperreflexic
4/4 = very hyperreflexic

- **DTR: 1/4 brachial B/L** (decreased reflex brachial DTR both sides)
- **DTR: R brachial & patella 4/4, L 2/4** (a patient who is hyperreflexic on one side of the body)

Gait

- Gait: **Ataxic** if unsteady. **Pt unable to walk** is fine if patient cannot walk.
- Romberg: **Positive** if patient cannot perform the test and falls to one side.

Meningeal Signs

- **Meningeal signs: + stiff neck, + Kernig, + Brudzinski**

Straight Leg Raising

- **Straight leg raise: positive R, neg on L** is how to chart the straight leg raise test.

Differential Diagnosis

One component of the Patient Note involves coming up with a Differential Diagnosis. This will also be asked of you for some patients on whom you have not done a physical exam. Guidelines for writing diagnoses include the following:

- Write the most likely diagnosis on the first line. You do get a little extra credit if you get the diagnosis correct on line #1.

- Do not use abbreviations on your diagnosis.

- Be as specific as possible. Congestive heart failure is correct, but SOB is not. In that case, no credit will be given.

- Use formal medical diagnoses. For example, "Panic disorder without agoraphobia" is correct, but "Anxiety" doesn't distinguish an actual medical diagnosis from something you might feel while taking Step 2 CS.

- Write diagnoses lower on the list only if they explain some of the patient's symptoms or physical findings.

- It is better to leave a couple of lines blank than to write down a diagnosis that has absolutely no support in the history and physical.

- Remember that "Noncompliance with medicine" or "Medication side effects" are legitimate diagnoses.

For each diagnosis you must list positive and/or negative findings that support your diagnosis. There is no set minimum number of history findings and physical exam findings stated. However, avoid leaving this section blank. You will be writing a lot of the same phrases here that you also used in the History and Physical sections of the note.

The test now requires you to give supporting information from the history and physical, both positives and negatives that support your diagnosis. It is helpful to have in mind a broad differential diagnosis for likely chief complaints and the kind of historical facts and physical exam elements that are likely to be on the grading checklists. Certainly you should have a differential in mind for sites of pain in all parts of the body, as well as common presenting complaints.

For a wide variety of examples of supporting documentation using the new exam format, refer to Appendix C: Differentials and Common Supporting Documentation for Assorted Chief Complaints.

Diagnostic Study

Another component of the Patient Note includes ordering the INITIAL workup on the patient. This component of the Patient Note is also required for surrogate and telephone cases, unless otherwise specified. The best approach to writing the Diagnostic Study is to follow a certain pattern; that way, you will not forget to document any important tests. Guidelines for writing the workup include the following:

- Make a habit of writing on the first line any prohibited physical exam maneuvers that the patient needs. For example, "Rectal exam with hemoccult" or "Complete physical exam."

- If you do not need to order any further physical exam maneuvers, go ahead and begin documenting diagnostic tests on the first line.

- Write on the first line any labs or x-rays that are needed now.

- First, order the simple baseline tests that the patient needs now.

- There are no mandates or rules about what line should have blood tests or what line should have x-rays. It does makes sense, however, to group things together as you do in real life. "CBC, lytes, glu, Cr, BUN."

- You should assume that all of the tests will be done now, at one time, unless you write otherwise.

- It is incorrect to write diagnostic tests on the same line as the particular diagnosis.

- The tests you do order should help support or exclude the diagnosis you are considering. For instance, if your only diagnosis is "trauma to the foot," it would be wrong to order pulmonary angiography, or screening colonoscopy.

- There is no cost containment on this test. In other words, graders are not looking for the single best test. However, there is harm to patients in ordering unnecessary tests, so be careful when you are ordering tests that might not be needed. Be especially careful when ordering tests that carry clear immediate harm, such as a CT scan, angiogram, or cardiac catheterization.

- If no testing is indicated (a rare event, but possible), simply write in this section, "No tests indicated."

Sample Cases

Case 1: **Ankle Pain**

DOORWAY INFORMATION

Opening Scenario

Mary Smith is a 21 y/o female who comes to the clinic complaining of ankle pain.

Vital Signs

- Temp: 38.3°C (101.0°F)
- BP: 120/80 mm Hg, right upper limb sitting
- HR: 80/min, regular
- RR: 20/min

Examinee Tasks

1. Obtain a focused history.
2. Perform a relevant physical examination. Do not perform rectal, pelvic, genitourinary, inguinal hernia, female breast, or corneal reflex examinations.
3. Discuss your initial diagnostic impression and your workup plan with the patient.
4. After leaving the room, complete your patient note on the given form.

BEFORE ENTERING THE ROOM

Clinical Reasoning: Consider listing several causes of ankle pain. Thinking about the diagnosis now allows you to do a more relevant history and focused physical. As with all musculoskeletal complaints, a history of trauma is key to guiding your approach. Consider the following conditions as part of your differential before you enter the room:

- Fracture
- Ligament injury
- Infection, e.g., Staph, gonococcal
- Deposition: crystals, gout

The HPI you obtain will help you quickly narrow down the list.

FROM THE STANDARDIZED PATIENT

History

HPI: Ms. Smith states that she twisted her right ankle one week ago when stepping off a curb. She felt a sudden popping sensation on the outside part of her right ankle. She scraped off a little skin from the outside of the ankle but had just a few drops of blood. The pain is severe and sharp, and it moves into her foot. She rates the pain as a 7/10 on the pain scale. Ms. Smith notices it is better when she elevates her leg and puts ice on the ankle. It hurts much worse when she walks on it, and she can walk only a couple of steps. In the last 3 days her right foot and ankle have been bothering her more, and she also noticed increasing redness and swelling in her right ankle with some oozing from the abrasion site. She has not noticed any fever. Before last week she never had any problems with her feet or ankles. She has missed classes for the last 3 days, as she takes public transportation to school. In addition, tennis season starts in 2 weeks and she is attending college on a tennis scholarship.

PMH: She has no allergies. She takes no medications. She has had no prior hospitalizations, trauma, major illness, or surgery.

Social Hx: She lives with her parents and denies any tobacco, alcohol, or drug use.

Physical Exam

Upon entering the room you notice that the patient is in obvious discomfort. She is holding her right ankle and foot. There is redness about the ankle joint, centered on the lateral malleolus. She is alert and cooperative, and her speech is normal.

Extremities: Inspection reveals normal L ankle. R ankle is red and swollen. No red streaking up the leg. There is also some red/purple discoloration under the lateral malleolus with small amount of discharge from small open wound. Palpation shows a nontender L ankle and very tender R lateral malleolus.

Normal range of motion on the L ankle. The R ankle has very limited ROM because of pain. She will not co-operate with strength testing at the R ankle because of pain. There is normal ROM in both knees. Left ankle strength (motor) is 5/5. Sensation to light touch is intact bilaterally. Dorsalis pedis and posterior tibial pulses are equal 2/4 bilaterally.

THE CLOSING

As with all cases, it is also important to explain to your patient your clinical impression and discuss the next steps in working up her condition. It is important to provide some indication about the length of time she may be unable to walk, as she has already let you know her concern about missing classes and being ready for tennis season. Be sure to answer any additional concerns she may have.

> **Doctor:** "I believe you may have a broken ankle. However, I am also considering the possibility of an infection in your ankle because of your fever. So that we can treat you appropriately, I am going to take a blood test to look for an infection and an x-ray picture of your ankle to look for a broken bone. I can do these tests right now, and then we can discuss the results and plan treatment. Do you have any questions?"

CHALLENGING QUESTIONS

Be prepared to answer the following types of challenging questions for this particular case:

Ms. Smith: "Is it fractured or is it just sprained?"

Doctor: "I will take a picture to find out if the bone is injured. It's possible that you may have injured or torn some of the ligaments in your ankle. Ligaments help keep the ankle stable. I understand how important it is to be able to get to class and play tennis for the school."

Ms. Smith: "I have a tennis scholarship for college. When do you think I'll be able to play again?"

Doctor: "When I have the x-ray, I will be better able to tell you the nature of the injury and when you might be able to play tennis."

SAMPLE PATIENT NOTE

History: Describe the history you just obtained from this patient. Include only information (pertinent positives and negatives) relevant to this patient's problem(s).

CC: "My ankle hurts."

HPI: R ankle pain maximum at lateral malleolus
        – Pain is severe, sharp, without radiation; 7/10 intensity
        – Began suddenly 1 week ago when stepping off a curb; twisted ankle and felt a "pop"
        – Also got abrasion to R lateral malleolus, now with redness and swelling
        – Denies fever, no prior episodes of ankle problems

Meds: None, NKDA

PMH: No hospitalizations, major illness, past trauma, surgery

SH: Lives with parents, denies tobacco, EtOH, or drug use

SAMPLE PATIENT NOTE

Physical Exam: Describe any positive and negative findings relevant to this patient's problem(s). Be careful to include only those parts of examination you performed in *this* encounter.

VS: NL except for T = 101.0°F

GA: In mild distress 2nd ankle pain

R Ankle: Swollen, red, tender over lateral malleolus. Some ecchymosis also present. Unable to check ROM, motor due to pain. No lymphangitis. Small open wound at lateral malleolus, discharge. No popliteal adenopathy bilaterally. Distal sensation intact.

L Ankle/Leg: NL skin, nontender, Full NL dorsiflexion, plantar flexion, eversion, inversion. Strength 5/5.

Ext: Pulses DP, PT 2/4 bilaterally. Light touch sensation intact both feet bilaterally.

SAMPLE PATIENT NOTE

Data Interpretation: *Based on what you have learned from the history and physical examination,* list up to 3 diagnoses that might explain this patient's complaint(s). List your diagnoses from most to least likely. For some cases, fewer than 3 diagnoses will be appropriate. Then, enter the positive or negative findings from the history and the physical examination (if present) that support each diagnosis. Lastly, list initial *diagnostic* studies (if any) you would order for this patient (e.g., restricted physical exam maneuvers, laboratory tests, imaging, ECG, etc.).

Diagnosis #1: Cellulitis of ankle

Differential diagnosis and diagnostic reasoning

History Finding(s)	Physical Exam Finding(s)
Abrasion 1 week ago	Fever
Increasing redness and swelling	Red and swollen
	Tender to touch
	Open wound with discharge

Diagnosis #2: Sprain of ankle

Differential diagnosis and diagnostic reasoning

History Finding(s)	Physical Exam Finding(s)
Twisted ankle and heard pop sound	Tender lateral ligament of ankle
	Decreased ROM

Diagnosis #3: Fracture of ankle

Differential diagnosis and diagnostic reasoning

History Finding(s)	Physical Exam Finding(s)
Twisted ankle and felt pop	Point tender at lateral malleolus
	Ecchymosis at ankle laterally

Diagnostic Study/Studies

X-ray R ankle

Wound C&S

CBC, blood C&S

CASE DISCUSSION

Notes about the History-Taking

For this case, it is best not to offer to shake the patient's hand during your introduction. This patient is in obvious pain and is preoccupied with using her hands to splint her painful ankle. The most appropriate step when first entering the room is to attend to the patient's comfort and offer support.

The initial history of stepping off a curb, twisting her ankle, and feeling a popping sensation is typical of an ankle sprain and/or fracture. However, it is important that you are able to recognize pertinent findings such as fever and the history of an abrasion. The abrasion, fever, and redness all suggest cellulitis.

When a traumatic injury interferes with ambulation, it's essential that you explore how this is impacting the patient's life, demonstrate empathy, and offer support.

Notes about the Physical Exam

The physical exam checklist highlights the importance of documenting the findings of both sides of any paired structures in the body. Had you documented physical exam findings on only one extremity, you would have missed about half of the physical exam checklist items. As a general rule, inspect and palpate at least one joint above and one joint below the site of injury. With a fall, injury is possible anywhere on the injured extremity and may be in more than one location. Specifically for the ankle, the lateral malleolus is most commonly injured from an inversion injury. Associated areas to palpate, because they are sometimes also injured, are both malleoli, the Achilles tendon, and the base of the 5th metatarsal, as well as the proximal fibula.

In this case the pain is so intense that the patient will not cooperate and move the ankle no matter how nicely you ask or how well you explain your intent. In most cases the patient will cooperate with physical exam maneuvers when you show empathy and explain their importance. If you have made two attempts to get a patient to cooperate with a physical exam maneuver and the patient still refuses, recognize that this is part of the case and simply move on to your next step in the physical examination.

Be sure to comment on any discolorations or skin markings you may observe, even if these markings are due to makeup (a technique used in order to simulate physical findings). In any patient with red-powdered skin, consider any diagnosis that includes inflammation and infection.

Checking for lymphangitis and enlarged popliteal or femoral nodes is important, in order to look for spread of the infection.

Comments about the Patient Note

All notes should contain a comment about the vital signs and general appearance. A common mistake on a case of an isolated extremity is to write only the physical exam of the injured extremity. It is essential to compare the good side to the bad, and include in your note the physical findings of the normal side as well.

Case 2: **Back Pain**

BEFORE ENTERING THE ROOM

Clinical Reasoning: Because there are many different causes of back pain, you will first need to determine the site of the back pain (cervical, thoracic, or lumbar). For all levels of the spine there may be a fracture, infection, tumor, disk disease, or paraspinal muscle pain. However, not all pain in the back is coming from the spine and musculoskeletal system. Knowing what organs cause pain in the back will be your cues for the organ systems you will ask about and examine.

FROM THE STANDARDIZED PATIENT

History

HPI: Mr. Jones states that his back hurts. The pain is located 2 inches to the right of the midline at the level of his belt. It is 3/10 pain if he is completely still. The pain increases to 7/10 on the pain scale with any movement or twisting. He had to call his neighbor to tie his shoes this morning, as he wasn't able to bend over without the sharp pain. It started a little bit last night after work but by morning it was really hard to get out of bed. He thought maybe he hurt it at work yesterday afternoon, as he felt a sudden twinge when picking up a car transmission by himself.

The patient took 2 aspirin right away and put some ice on his back as soon as he felt the pain yesterday. He was able to finish the workday. "No work, no pay," Mr. Jones explains. He felt a little better after the aspirin but not back to normal. The pain sometimes is just in his back and sometimes radiates into his side of his thigh but not past his knee. He denies any pain, numbness, or weakness in the legs. There has been no incontinence of stool or urine. Mr. Jones denies any numbness in the genitals. He has had no fevers and no recent weight loss.

He has had back pain only once before, when he had a kidney stone 5 years ago. He states that pain was worse with the kidney stone because he could not find a comfortable position. Today the pain is bearable if he is completely still.

PMH: He has no history of malignancies. He has no allergies. He takes no medications other than an occasional ASA for a headache and has never taken steroids. He was hospitalized once, at age 18 for appendicitis. No traumatic injuries other than a sprained ankle in high school once. Denies diabetes and hypertension.

Family Hx: No family members with chronic back pain.

Social Hx: Divorced, lives alone with two large dogs. Denies any tobacco, alcohol, or IV drug use. Works as an auto mechanic. His only stress is worrying about missing work and the mess the dogs are going to make if he doesn't get home soon.

Physical Exam

Upon entering the room, you notice that the patient is in obvious discomfort. He is standing up, perfectly still, at the side of the exam table, bent slightly forward at the waist. His right hand is holding his sore back and his left hand is on the exam table to steady himself. Mr. Jones is alert and cooperative verbally but doesn't want to sit down. His breathing is normal. Lungs are clear to auscultation. Respiratory excursion is normal. Heart sounds are normal without murmur or rub. Inspection of his back shows no bruising or erythema. Palpation of the spinous process in the cervical, thoracic, and lumbar area are nontender. Palpation of the right paraspinal muscles at about T12–L4 is very tender and reproduces the pain. His gait is very slow, with small steps, as his back hurts. He has very limited ROM in the lumbar spine because of pain. There is no CVA tenderness bilaterally.

With great coaxing, the patient agrees to lie down on the exam table if you pull out the footstool and help him. The abdomen is soft, with bowel sounds present. No masses or tenderness. Extremities are without deformity or rash. Plantarflexion, dorsiflexion of the foot, and lower leg strength are all normal and equal bilaterally. Patella and Achilles reflexes are intact, 2/4 bilaterally. Sensation to light touch is intact just above the kneecap, over the lateral lower leg, and over the lateral aspect of the foot bilaterally. Straight leg raise is negative bilaterally. Dorsalis pedis and posterior tibial pulses are normal bilaterally.

THE CLOSING

As with all cases, it's important to explain your clinical impression to the patient and discuss the next steps in working up his condition. It's also important to speak about how he can get some assistance with daily activities for a couple of days. Be sure to answer any additional concerns he may have.

CHALLENGING QUESTIONS

Be prepared to answer the following type of challenging question for this case:

Mr. Jones: "Do I have a herniated disk? Might I need an MRI?"

Doctor: "It's possible that you could have a herniated disk, but I'm not finding any evidence of that. You have no worrisome symptoms or physical exam signs that would indicate pressure on the spine or nerves coming off the spine, so an MRI isn't indicated right now. I believe you most likely have a painful back strain. This might take a couple of days to get better. Do you have anyone who can help with walking the dogs?"

SAMPLE PATIENT NOTE

History: Describe the history you just obtained from this patient. Include only information (pertinent positives and negatives) relevant to this patient's problem(s).

CC: Back pain

HPI: Sharp pain in the R lower back, 3/10 intensity at rest, 7/10 with any movement. Began yesterday when lifting a "transmission." Somewhat relieve by OTC meds yesterday but pain much worse this morning. Some radiation to thighs but never below level of the knee. No weakness or numbness. No perineal paresthesia or incontinence. No blood in the urine. No fever or weight loss.

PMH: Hospitalized for appy at age 18 and had kidney stone 5 years ago. No trauma. No history of malignancies, IVDU

Meds: None, never used steroids

FH: No chronic back pain in family

SH: Lives alone with two dogs. No alcohol, drugs, or tobacco. Works as mechanic.

SAMPLE PATIENT NOTE

Physical Exam: Describe any positive and negative findings relevant to this patient's problem(s). Be careful to include *only* those parts of examination you performed in *this* encounter.

VS: WNL

GA: In distress secondary to lower back pain. Pt standing still, slightly bent over in pain. Pt is holding his back with his hand.

Inspection: No skin change, no bruise, no deformity.

Back: No point tenderness in spinal processes cervical, thoracic, or lumbar. No CVA tenderness. Very tender R lumbar paraspinal muscle at lower thoracic and upper lumbar level.

Abd: Soft, BS+, no masses or tenderness

Neuro: L4, L5, S1 Motor intact 5/5 lower ext B/L
            L4, L5, S1 Light touch sensation intact B/L
            Achilles, patellar reflex 2/4 B/L
            Straight leg raise negative B/L

Pulse: 2/4 DP, PT B/L

SAMPLE PATIENT NOTE

Data Interpretation: *Based on what you have learned from the history and physical examination,* list up to 3 diagnoses that might explain this patient's complaint(s). List your diagnoses from most to least likely. For some cases, fewer than 3 diagnoses will be appropriate. Then, enter the positive or negative findings from the history and the physical examination (if present) that support each diagnosis. Lastly, list initial *diagnostic* studies (if any) you would order for this patient (e.g., restricted physical exam maneuvers, laboratory tests, imaging, ECG, etc.).

Diagnosis #1: Muscle strain of back

Differential diagnosis and diagnostic reasoning

History Finding(s)	Physical Exam Finding(s)
Sudden pain with lifting	R paraspinal muscles tender
No leg weakness, numbness	Normal distal motor in legs
No hematuria	Normal distal ankle, knee reflex
No colicky pain	Negative straight leg raise

Diagnosis #2: Herniated disk

Differential diagnosis and diagnostic reasoning

History Finding(s)	Physical Exam Finding(s)
Back pain with radiation to thigh only	Normal distal motor, sensory
	Negative straight leg raise

Diagnosis #3: Fracture of spine

Differential diagnosis and diagnostic reasoning

History Finding(s)	Physical Exam Finding(s)
Severe pain lifting heavy object	Area near spinous process tender
Worse with movement	

Diagnostic Study/Studies

Rectal exam to check tone

CASE DISCUSSION

Notes about the History-Taking

This man has a back strain by history and physical, a very common ailment. Some patients with back pain find that standing or lying flat provides some relief and is better than sitting. It is perfectly fine to take the history while the patient stands. It is important to overtly acknowledge the patient's discomfort and express empathy.

Your introduction might go something like this:

> **Doctor:** "Hello. I'm Dr. First-Name Last-Name. I will be your physician today. I see you're in a lot of pain. Would you be more comfortable lying down? I can help."
>
> **Mr. Jones:** "I'd rather stand, Doc."
>
> **Doctor:** "Sure, that's fine. Tell me all about what happened."

The fact that the pain began when the patient lifted something very heavy, and the fact that he wants to stand perfectly still, both indicate a musculoskeletal problem. With a history of back pain, it is important to assess all "red flags."

- Ask about pain, paresthesia, and weakness in the legs.
- Patients with bowel or bladder incontinence, decreased rectal tone, and paresthesias of the perineum or urinary retention may have cauda equina syndrome.
- Ask about history of cancer, immunosuppression, and past steroid use.
- Ask about fever, unexplained weight loss, and IV drug use.

The key to assessing for radiculopathy/nerve root compression is determining whether the pain radiates in the sciatic distribution. This is most significant if the pain radiates all the way to the foot, not just to the thigh.

The social history is important in any case where the illness is possibly affecting the patient's ability to dress, eat, ambulate, toilet, and perform hygiene on his own.

Notes about the Physical Exam

Since the chief complaint is back pain, it's best to start with the back exam. That way, if you're short on time you can be sure you have completed an important step on the checklist. During palpation, be sure to palpate the midline and spinous processes separately from the CVA areas and the paraspinal areas. A meticulous physical can save a lot of unnecessary tests and, more importantly, gets you an accurate diagnosis. Detailed testing of the L4, L5, S1 nerve-root motor, sensory, and reflex will be on every checklist that possibly has sciatica as a potential diagnosis.

Understanding the correct procedure for and interpretation of the straight leg raise is key. With the patient lying flat and the knee fully extended, slowly flex the hip from 180° to 90°. A positive test occurs when the patient describes pain radiating in the sciatic distribution down the leg. It should be exacerbated with dorsiflexion of the foot.

Comments about the Patient Note

Did you want to get a spine x-ray on Mr. Jones? He is young, without osteoporosis, and he did not fall or have direct trauma, such as being hit with a baseball bat. He has no fever, no drug use, no steroids, and no sciatica symptoms or neurological deficits. The yield of significant findings on x-ray in this population is very low.

The patient is worried about a herniated disk and requesting an MRI. Know the current guidelines, which do not recommend MRI for patients with acute low back pain but no red flags on history and no neurological deficits on physical exam.

The rectal tone exam was requested just to rule out an injury to the spinal cord or nerve roots.

Case 3: **Sore Throat**

BEFORE ENTERING THE ROOM

Clinical Reasoning: Consider the following conditions as part of your differential before you enter the room:

- Pharyngitis
- Upper respiratory infection
- Infection, e.g., bacterial (Strep), viral
- Epiglottitis
- Peritonsillar abscess

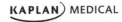

FROM THE STANDARIZED PATIENT

History

HPI: Ms. Johnson has had a severe sore throat for 1 week. She describes it as 8/10 in intensity, and it is very painful to swallow, even her own saliva. She has felt feverish and sluggish for the past week. She has not taken her temperature. She feels like she has no energy. Tylenol makes her feel slightly better for a few hours and she can sip some water or tea. Nothing seems to make it worse. It has been difficult for her to go to ice hockey practice even though she is team captain. Ms. Johnson has no cough or sputum and no shortness of breath. She states she has had decreased appetite and lost 2–3 lb. because it hurts when she swallows. She complains that her neck seems swollen. She has been sleeping more than usual. Her roommate was diagnosed with Strep throat last month. Her boyfriend is not ill.

PMH: She is allergic to penicillin. She was just a child when she first received it, but she remembers that it gave her a very itchy and lumpy rash all over. She takes no medications. She has had no prior hospitalizations, trauma, major illness, or surgery.

Ob/Gyn: LMP was 2 weeks ago and normal. She has a boyfriend but is not sexually active.

Social Hx: She lives in her college dormitory with her roommate. She denies any tobacco, alcohol, or recreational drug use.

Physical Exam

Upon entering the room you notice that patient is in obvious discomfort. She winces when she swallows. There is no rash or skin discoloration. Her head is normocephalic and atraumatic. Her sclera are clear and not jaundiced. Her pupils are equal, round, reactive to light. Tympanic membranes are normal. Nares are without congestion. Pharynx is red and inflamed. No exudates. Tonsils are enlarged. She has diffuse adenopathy, most prominent in the posterior cervical lymph nodes. Neck is supple. Her anterior neck hurts when the lymph glands are palpated. Lungs are clear to auscultation. Heart auscultation is normal. Her abdomen appears normal. She has tenderness in the abdomen just below the left costal margin upon palpation. Her spleen is not palpable. Bowel sounds are present. She is alert and oriented to person, place, and time. Her gait is normal.

THE CLOSING

As with all cases, explain your clinical impression to the patient and discuss the next steps in working up her condition. It is important to provide some counseling about how her illness will affect her role as hockey captain. Be sure to answer any additional concerns she may have.

> **Doctor:** "On your physical exam I saw that your throat is very red, you have a little fever, and there is some tenderness in your belly. I think you could have an infection in your throat. I'd like to take a throat swab to check. Also, I'd like to take a blood test to check for mono." *(Most college students know what mono is, so likely no definition is needed.)* "Then we will discuss the results. Once we know what kind of infection you have, we'll know how to treat it."

CHALLENGING QUESTIONS

Be prepared to answer the following challenging question:

Patient: "If I have mono, what does that mean for ice hockey?"

Doctor: "If you have mono, it's possible that your spleen could be swollen. The risk of serious injury might mean you have to keep away from contact sports for a few weeks."

SAMPLE PATIENT NOTE

History: Describe the history you just obtained from this patient. Include only information (pertinent positives and negatives) relevant to this patient's problem(s).

CC: Sore throat

HPI: • Severe sore throat for 1 wk, difficulty swallowing, front of neck feels swollen.
            8/10 intensity, no radiation. Better with Tylenol, nothing makes it worse.
          • Positive: 1 wk of feeling feverish, tired
            Negative: cough, coryza, SOB, or sputum
            Roommate recently treated for Strep throat

Meds: None. Allergic to PCN with generalized itching.

PMH: No hospitalizations, major illness, trauma, surgery
          LMP: 2 wks ago, NL

SX: Not sexually active

SHx: Lives in college dorm. Denies tobacco, EtOH, or drug use.

SAMPLE PATIENT NOTE

Physical Examination: Describe any positive and negative findings relevant to this patient's problem(s). Be careful to include *only* those parts of examination you performed in this encounter.

VS: NL except for T = 101.7°F

GA: NAD

HEENT: Pharynx red with swollen tonsils. Airway intact. Uvula midline. TMs, nares NL. PERRL.

Neck: Supple, diffusely tender cervical adenopathy

Lungs: Clear to auscultation

Abd: Soft, with tenderness in the RUQ, no masses or rebound. Spleen not palpable.

SAMPLE PATIENT NOTE

Data Interpretation: *Based on what you have learned from the history and physical examination,* list up to 3 diagnoses that might explain this patient's complaint(s). List your diagnoses from most to least likely. For some cases, fewer than 3 diagnoses will be appropriate. Then, enter the positive or negative findings from the history and the physical examination (if present) that support each diagnosis. Lastly, list initial *diagnostic* studies (if any) you would order for this patient (e.g., restricted physical exam maneuvers, laboratory tests, imaging, ECG, etc.).

Diagnosis #1: Mononucleosis

Differential diagnosis and diagnostic reasoning

History Finding(s)	**Physical Exam Finding(s)**
1 week feeling tired	Erythema of pharynx
Sore throat	Diffuse neck adenopathy
Swollen neck	Tender liver
Feverish	

Diagnosis #2: Strep pharyngitis

Differential diagnosis and diagnostic reasoning

History Finding(s)	**Physical Exam Finding(s)**
Sore throat	Fever
Exposure to Strep	Erythema of pharynx
No coryza	Tender lymphadenopathy
Feverish feeling	

Diagnosis #3: Peritonsillar abscess

Differential diagnosis and diagnostic reasoning

History Finding(s)	**Physical Exam Finding(s)**
Sore throat	Fever
Difficulty swallowing own saliva	Erythema of pharynx, uvula midline
	No trismus

Diagnostic Study/Studies

CBC

Mono spot

Throat culture

T. bili, ALT, AST

CASE DISCUSSION

Notes about the History-Taking

At the doorway you should begin thinking of a differential diagnosis for sore throat. In addition to the differentials listed in this case, you can also consider:

- Adult epiglottitis, which causes a severe sore throat accompanied by a very hoarse voice
- Peritonsillar abscess, which presents with a severe sore throat and trismus. Trismus is the inability to open the mouth completely
- Upper respiratory infection
- Allergic rhinitis, the absence of coryza making it much less likely that the patient has this condition

Ms. Johnson's lack of energy or sluggish feeling associated with the sore throat could be a clue that this is a mononucleosis case.

Asking about exposure to Strep throat is an additional standard question frequently asked of patients who present with sore throat. The social history of living in a college dormitory, which typically has crowded conditions, can often be included in cases of other infectious diseases such as influenza, meningococcemia, or even TB.

Notes about the Physical Exam

The physical exam checklist highlights the importance of recognizing that a temperature of 100.4°F or greater represents a fever case. The fever of 101.7°F in a young adult increases the likelihood of a bacterial or more serious viral infection. The focused physical exam concentrates on the organ systems involved. So for pharyngitis, a fairly complete HEENT exam is needed. Whenever you are considering an upper respiratory infection (URI), an exam for a lower respiratory tract infection (pneumonia) is also indicated. Since this patient has had no pulmonary symptoms (cough, sputum, or SOB, for instance), auscultation is sufficient.

Mononucleosis causes hepatosplenomegaly, which in this case is causing her abdominal tenderness to palpation. Even though Ms. Johnson does not complain of abdominal pain, an abdominal exam is still indicated with complaint of sore throat in a younger person, in order to look for this possibility.

Since the patient is in some distress with extreme difficulty swallowing, caution must be used when examining the pharynx. In adults epiglottitis rarely causes airway obstruction, but with younger children or adolescents this can be a concern. If a patient says they can't easily open their mouth, take this as a hint and only gently see if they can allow examination of their pharynx. When considering peritonsillar abscess, it's important to note position of the uvula and absence of trismus.

Liver function tests (LFTs) were obtained because most patients with mononucleosis have some elevation in their liver enzymes. Ordering LFTs would be mandatory if she also mentioned skin yellowing, or if she had yellow makeup dabbed on her as a simulated physical finding. Finally, a throat culture was ordered in this case. A Strep screen would also have been correct.

Case 4: **Car Accident**

DOORWAY INFORMATION

Opening Scenario

Bill Rodgers is a 59 y/o male brought to you at the hospital after having been in a car accident.

Vital Signs

- Temp: 37.0°C (98.6°F)
- BP: 160/90 mm Hg
- HR: 110/min, irregular
- RR: 20/min

Examinee Tasks

1. Obtain a focused history.
2. Perform a relevant physical examination. Do not perform rectal, pelvic, genitourinary, inguinal hernia, female breast, or corneal reflex examinations.
3. Discuss your initial diagnostic impression and your workup plan with the patient.
4. After leaving the room, complete your patient note on the given form.

BEFORE ENTERING THE ROOM

Clinical Reasoning: The challenge in this case is to obtain a history but to then focus most of your attention on the physical examination. The physical exam for acute trauma emphasizes inspection and palpation of all areas of the body. On a blunt trauma case you will need to inspect and palpate each section of the body to see if there are any "hidden" bruises or fractures. Rapidly palpate each extremity in two or three places with your open hand. If you are close to a simulated physical finding, the patient will grimace and then you can slow down and determine exactly where the injury is located. Pay attention to all information on the doorway.

FROM THE STANDARDIZED PATIENT

History

HPI: Mr. Rodgers was not wearing his seat belt when his car was hit from behind 30 minutes ago. Mr. Rodgers says he was stopped at a red light when this happened. He doesn't really remember the accident, and the first thing he can recall afterward is waking up with a sore neck while the paramedics were knocking on the window. Mr. Rodgers quickly regained consciousness and then unlocked the door. The neck pain is described as sharp, 5/10 intensity. He states that pain is worse when he tries to bend his neck, and better if he keeps perfectly still. He has no prior neck problems or any other injury, nor does he have any chest pain, shortness of breath, abdominal pain, or problems with his extremities.

PMH: Patient is allergic to strawberries. He was started on warfarin and metoprolol 1 week ago after having new-onset palpitations for which he was diagnosed with atrial fibrillation. He has never had any surgery or other trauma. He has had a history of hypertension for 20 years for which he takes lisinopril.

Social Hx: Mr. Rodgers has smoked one pack of cigarettes a day for the last 20 years. He has not had any alcohol for the past week, as he was advised to eliminate his daily glass of wine with dinner. He lives with his wife.

Physical Exam

The patient is alert and oriented to person, place, and time. He comes in walking normally, rubbing his neck. He has an obvious purple/blue ecchymosis to the forehead. The skin is intact. There is no deformity to the calvarium. PEERL. Pharynx and nares are normal. There is no hemotympanum. His neck is tender in the midline posteriorly as well as in both trapezius bilaterally. His chest is normal-appearing, and he has a normal respiratory excursion. Palpation of the chest wall reveals no tenderness or deformity. Radial pulses are 2/4 and equal bilaterally. Lungs are clear to auscultation. Heart tones are irregular without murmur. The abdomen is soft and nontender in all quadrants. No ecchymosis or abrasions present. There is no CVA tenderness.

His extremities are free of any trauma. He has no facial asymmetry, CN 9, 10, 12 are also intact. His motor strength is 5/5 all four extremities.

THE CLOSING

The closings seem more artificial the sicker the patient is portraying. Even had this been a multiple trauma case with life-threatening injuries, you would still do the closing. Remember, there is no treatment in Step 2 CS.

> **Doctor:** "Mr. Rodgers, I have completed your physical exam and I would like to tell you what I'm thinking. First of all, let me be sure I understand. You started warfarin recently for abnormal heartbeat, and today you bumped your head and hurt your neck in a car accident. Is that correct?" *(Wait for the response)*
>
> "On your physical exam I see a bruise on your forehead, and your neck seems pretty sore. You most likely have a sprained neck, but I will ask you to have an x-ray to be sure. I will also take a picture of your head, and a blood test to check the warfarin level. As soon as the x-ray is completed, I'll come and tell you the results. Do you have any questions?"

CHALLENGING QUESTIONS

Mr. Rodgers: "I should have taken my warfarin a half-hour ago. May I take my own tablet? I have it with me."

Doctor: "Please wait and let's get a picture of your head first. Then I'll know if you should take it or not."

Any patient who wants medication for any reason should always get the same response: You always need to do a history and physical, do a test, and then you'll know the correct medicine to give.

SAMPLE PATIENT NOTE

History: Describe the history you just obtained from this patient. Include only information (pertinent positives and negatives) relevant to this patient's problem(s).

CC: MVA (motor vehicle accident)

HPI: Patient states he was rear-ended in the car 30 minutes ago while stopped at red light. No seat belt. Refused paramedic help and insisted on walking into hospital himself. Neck pain is sharp/burning feeling, 5/10 intensity. Radiates to both shoulders bilaterally. Better with rest. Hurts with any movement of the neck. Denies chest pain, SOB, Abd pain, or extremity pain. Denies any weakness in the extremities. Also states had brief LOC as he hit his head.

Allergies: Strawberries

Medications: Warfarin (1 wk), metoprolol (1 wk), lisinopril

PMH: No prior trauma. Hospitalized for first presentation of sustained atrial fibrillation last week, and started on the medication. Hx of HTN as well. No surgical hx.

SH: States drank 1 glass of wine per day but stopped on advice of cardiologist last week. Still smokes 1 pack of cigarettes/day. Lives at home with his wife.

SAMPLE PATIENT NOTE

Physical Examination: Describe any positive and negative findings relevant to this patient's problem(s). Be careful to include *only* those parts of examination you performed in *this* encounter.

VS: HR 110 and irreg, BP 160/90, T 37.0°C, RR 20

GA: Awake, alert, mild distress, complaining of neck pain

HEENT: Contusion and tenderness to forehead. No laceration. PERRL. TMs clear. Pharynx: clear, no other facial bone tenderness.

Cervical spine: Tender in the midline and both trapezius bilaterally. No thoracic, lumbar, or CVA tenderness.

Chest: No bruising, NL respiratory excursion. No chest wall tenderness. Lungs clear to A.

CV: S1 S2 WNL no RMG, radial pulses strong and irregular, 2/4 B/L.

Abd: Nontender

Ext: No tenderness to palpation all 4 ext

Neuro: Alert and oriented to person, place, and time. No facial asymmetry. Motor 5/5 all 4 ext. Gait intact.

SAMPLE PATIENT NOTE

Data Interpretation: Based on what you have learned from the history and physical examination, list up to 3 diagnoses that might explain this patient's complaint(s). List your diagnoses from most to least likely. For some cases, fewer than 3 diagnoses will be appropriate. Then, enter the positive or negative findings from the history and the physical examination (if present) that support each diagnosis. Lastly, list initial diagnostic studies (if any) you would order for this patient (e.g., restricted physical exam maneuvers, laboratory tests, imaging, ECG, etc.).

Diagnosis #1: Acute cervical strain

Differential diagnosis and diagnostic reasoning

History Finding(s)	Physical Exam Finding(s)
Pain in neck after MVA	Tender postcervical muscles
Pain worse with movement	Normal distal neuro exam

Diagnosis #2: Cervical vertebrae fracture

Differential diagnosis and diagnostic reasoning

History Finding(s)	Physical Exam Finding(s)
Pain in neck after MVA	Tender post c-spine in midline
Pain worse with movement	

Diagnosis #3: Intracranial hemorrhage

Differential diagnosis and diagnostic reasoning

History Finding(s)	Physical Exam Finding(s)
Blunt head trauma	Bruise on head
+ LOC	Tender forehead
On warfarin	

Diagnostic Study/Studies

CBC, INR

C-spine x-ray

CT of brain

ECG

CASE DISCUSSION

Notes about the History-Taking

This case is primarily designed to test your skills in handling a trauma patient. There are other elements in the history that in a normal office visit would require more thorough questioning. The possible neck injury and/or other possible injuries (fractures or bleeding) are the most important problems to address.

Notes about the Physical Exam

In this case, it would be incorrect (and potentially dangerous) to check the neck's range of motion prior to x-ray. In an ordinary emergency room setting you would provide immediate treatment with a cervical collar and c-spine immobilization. However, the Step 2 CS exam does not test your management and treatment skills; instead, you are tested on your clinical reasoning skills relating to the history and physical examination. Offer to help by holding the patient's head and neck still to prevent pain while the patient is lying down or changing position. Try not to move the neck throughout the entire encounter. Providing assistance to the SP during the encounter shows concern for the patient, and he will appreciate that you have helped to prevent the sharp pain that occurs when he moves his neck.

Note that in a case such as this you may or may not find the SP to have an irregular pulse from chronic atrial fibrillation. Be sure to check the radial pulse for 3–5 seconds to determine if it is regular or not.

Comments about the Patient Note

You may document the loss of consciousness at the very beginning of the HPI. What's important is that you have documented *both* the neck pain and the loss of consciousness. Where exactly you document the loss of consciousness (LOC) in the HPI narrative is less important.

Checking the INR on this patient, who is on warfarin, is mandatory. Anyone with even a brief loss of consciousness needs a head CT to look for bleeding inside the skull. In this case, write Epidural and Subdural on one line of the diagnosis. Using two separate lines is equally correct.

Atrial fibrillation did not make the list of top 3 diagnoses. Focus on the reason for today's visit with the doctor: the car accident. The a-fib is old news. Of course, getting the history of being on warfarin is important.

Case 5: **Left Arm Weakness**

BEFORE ENTERING THE ROOM

Clinical Reasoning: Left arm weakness can have many causes. Nervous system, vascular (blood flow), and musculoskeletal problems are all possible causes of weakness. A detailed examination of the arm, with close attention to motor strength, range of motion, and distal pulse, is an important part of this case. The weakness may also be coming from the spinal cord or nerve roots. Lastly, stroke is a common cause of weakness and should always be considered in an older patient. Be sure to include other questions about stroke in your history. Before you enter the room you will already be able to anticipate that a complete neurological exam will be needed in this patient.

FROM THE STANDARDIZED PATIENT

History

HPI: Mr. King presents to the ER and tells you that about an hour ago he started to have problems moving his left arm. He is right-handed. He was sitting at his computer typing when it started. When he got up and walked, he noticed that his left leg was dragging a bit.

The deficit came on pretty suddenly over the course of a couple of minutes. It now is getting neither better nor worse. Mr. King is getting worried that something bad is happening, as he could not put on and button his own jacket when he left for the emergency room. He took an aspirin tablet, but that doesn't seem to help. Nothing makes it worse. He has also noticed that he has trouble swallowing, and his face seems droopy. He almost choked while getting down the aspirin and a little water. He has no chest pain, headache, nausea, vomiting, or recent palpitations over the last few days.

He has never had anything this severe before, but last week his left arm got a little weak and numb but it only lasted several hours. Mr. King dismissed it as just being a little tired.

Allergies: None

Meds: HCTZ, lisinopril, ASA, Plavix, metoprolol, Lipitor

PMH: He was hospitalized for aortofemoral bypass surgery 1 year ago for claudication. He had a heart attack 2 years ago and had angioplasty with a stent performed. No diabetes or history of stroke. No trauma. Mr. King has a 5-year history of hypertension.

Social Hx: He has been sleeping normally; is trying unsuccessfully to eat a low-cholesterol, low-fat diet; and has no problems urinating.

He lives with his wife of 48 years; she is disabled and he is responsible for taking care of all of her needs, including feeding and toileting. Mr. King stopped smoking years ago. He has one shot of whiskey every Sunday afternoon.

Physical Exam

Patient appears somewhat sloppily dressed, and his left shoelace is untied. He prefers to look to the right. He has some droopiness to the left-lower face. His forehead is wrinkled, and he can close his eyes when asked. He has normal carotid artery pulses and no bruits. His chest appears normal. His breathing is normal and his lungs are clear. He has normal regular heart tones. Pulse is regular. He is alert and oriented to person, place, and time. He has difficulty looking to the left. His pupils are equal, round, and reactive to light. The fundi show a normal red reflex. He has left temporal and right nasal visual field loss.

His motor strength is significantly weaker on the left side of the body than the right. His left arm is weaker than his left leg. He has decreased reflexes on the left patellar and brachial compared to the right. His gait is difficult because of the unilateral weakness. He has decreased sensation in the left upper and lower extremities.

THE CLOSING

Doctor: "On your exam, I see that your strength is decreased on one side. What you could have is a lack of blood going to your brain. I'd like to order an imaging test of your head to find out why this is happening. As soon as we have these tests back I can figure out the best treatment options for you."

CHALLENGING QUESTIONS

Mr. King: "Someone has to take care of my wife while I am here. She is helpless on her own."

Doctor: "Yes, I can have the social worker come speak to you and your family about what arrangements can be made while you are here. Is there a family member we should call now?"

SAMPLE PATIENT NOTE

History: Describe the history you just obtained from this patient. Include only information (pertinent positives and negatives) relevant to this patient's problem(s).

CC: Weakness LUE

HPI: R-handed patient began experiencing L arm and leg weakness 1 hour ago. Started suddenly. Not improving. This is the second episode like this. Last week had L arm numbness and weakness for several hours. Today has also noticed problems with vision and trouble swallowing. Before coming to ER had difficulty dressing himself. Took ASA without relief. No headache, nausea, vomiting, or chest pain. He lives with and is sole caretaker of wife who is bedridden.

Allergies: None

Meds: ASA, Plavix, Lipitor, metoprolol, lisinopril, HCTZ

PMH: Hospitalized for aortobifemoral bypass 1 yr ago. AMI 2 yrs ago with stent. No trauma, stroke, or DM. + HTN.

SH: Stopped smoking years ago. Has one shot of whiskey every Sunday afternoon.

SAMPLE PATIENT NOTE

Physical Examination: Describe any positive and negative findings relevant to this patient's problem(s). Be careful to include *only* those parts of examination you performed in *this* encounter.

VS: BP 160/110 mm Hg, HR 80/min and regular, RR 20/min, afebrile

GA: Pt appears in distress due to weakness. Shoe is untied on L.

HEENT: PEERL. Fundi: red reflex intact. Pt gaze is to the R with both eyes. Visual field L temporal & R nasal loss.

Chest: Lungs CTA

CV: S1 S2 WNL regular, no murmur. Carotid upstroke NL, no bruit. Radial 2/4 B/L. PT, DP 1/4 B/L, feet warm.

Neuro: Alert and oriented ×3
L lower face droopy
Motor RUE 5/5, RLE 5/5, LUE 2/5, LLE 3/5
DTR: R brachial, patellar 2/4. L brachial, patellar 1/4.
Sensory: Decrease light touch LUE, LLE side of face.
Gait: Difficult with leg weakness, no ataxia

SAMPLE PATIENT NOTE

Data Interpretation: *Based on what you have learned from the history and physical examination,* list up to 3 diagnoses that might explain this patient's complaint(s). List your diagnoses from most to least likely. For some cases, fewer than 3 diagnoses will be appropriate. Then, enter the positive or negative findings from the history and the physical examination (if present) that support each diagnosis. Lastly, list initial *diagnostic* studies (if any) you would order for this patient (e.g., restricted physical exam maneuvers, laboratory tests, imaging, ECG, etc.).

Diagnosis #1: Acute cerebral vascular accident

Differential diagnosis and diagnostic reasoning

History Finding(s)	Physical Exam Finding(s)
1 hr left-sided weakness	L side 2/5–3/5 weak
History of vascular disease	Sensory deficit to light touch on left
Possible TIA last week	Left-sided neglect
	New facial droop
	Reflexes decreased on left brachial, patellar compared to right
	Homonymous hemianopia

Diagnosis #2: Transient ischemic attack

Differential diagnosis and diagnostic reasoning

History Finding(s)	Physical Exam Finding(s)
1 hr left-sided weakness	L side 2/5–3/5 weak
History of vascular disease	New facial droop
Possible TIA last week	Homonymous hemianopia

Diagnosis #3:

Differential diagnosis and diagnostic reasoning

History Finding(s)	Physical Exam Finding(s)

Diagnostic Study/Studies

Head CT (noncontrast)

CBC, lytes, BUN, Cr, glucose, INR

ECG, CXR

Carotid duplex scanning

CASE DISCUSSION

Notes about the History-Taking

Mr. King gives you the history that he has vascular disease. Since he has known peripheral vascular disease and known coronary artery disease, it is not surprising that he had a transient ischemic attack (TIA) last week and today is having either another TIA or a stroke. It is important to ask about headache, since headaches are more common in hemorrhagic stroke than ischemic stroke. You still need neuroimaging to confirm that a stroke is ischemic or hemorrhagic.

This patient would be an extreme emergency, as he may be a candidate for thrombolytic therapy.

The social history that Mr. King is the sole caretaker of his wife presents an additional problem. You'll need to address this during the closing. It is appropriate to offer to send a social worker to check on the wife and make arrangements for her care while Mr. King is with you.

Notes about the Physical Exam

The physical exam in this case concentrates on the neurological exam. In this case, there should be some testing of mental status, cranial nerves, motor, sensation, reflexes, and cerebellar function. Certainly, checking the carotid artery, auscultation of the heart, and lungs will complete the checklist.

Comments about the Patient Note

While this man probably has a right middle cerebral artery stroke, the important thing for Step 2 CS is to recognize the need for a good neurological exam and CNS workup. Be as specific as possible if you recognize a stroke syndrome. In this case, it's important to note that the pulse is regular, since so many strokes are from atrial fibrillation.

Patients with middle cerebral artery stroke tend to look toward the side of the brain that has the lesion, and tend to ignore the side of the body that is weak. (Notice that this patient had untied shoelaces on his left side.)

It is important to note that a CT scan was ordered in the workup plan as this patient will need imaging to determine whether they qualify for thrombolytic therapy. An MRI shows acute ischemia much sooner than CT, but a CT scan is more accurate in determining if an acute hemorrhage has occurred. While your inclination in this case might be to order a neurology consultation, Step 2 CS discourages relying on physicians for a recommended plan.

Case 6: **Nosebleed**

DOORWAY INFORMATION

Opening Scenario

Kevin Green is a 45 y/o male with a nosebleed.

Vital Signs

- Temp: 36.8°C (98.2°F)
- BP: 110/80 mm Hg
- HR: 88/min, regular
- RR: 18/min

Examinee Tasks

1. Obtain a focused history.
2. Perform a relevant physical examination. Do not perform rectal, pelvic, genitourinary, inguinal hernia, female breast, or corneal reflex examinations.
3. Discuss your initial diagnostic impression and your workup plan with the patient.
4. After leaving the room, complete your patient note on the given form.

BEFORE ENTERING THE ROOM

Clinical Reasoning: With a bleeding case, always consider three things:

- Patient's hemodynamic status
- Patient's ability to clot
- Underlying disease that may cause bleeding

With someone who has blood loss, it's important to check the hemodynamic status. Is the patient tachycardic? Does the Doorway Information show that he has a low blood pressure or a narrow pulse pressure?

The other thing you know is that a detailed examination to look for the source and type of bleeding is needed. Typically, dry air, nose-picking, and trauma can cause a bloody nose. Less common causes include polyps, allergies, and upper respiratory infections. Asking about cocaine is also relevant.

Finally, anyone presenting with bleeding as the primary problem might have a bleeding disorder. Be sure to inquire into the family history for diseases such as hemophilia or von Willebrand disease. Also, is the patient taking aspirin, warfarin, or any other medication or herbal products (e.g., ginkgo biloba) that can interfere with clotting? Does he have bone marrow failure? Perhaps the patient has liver disease and a coagulopathy?

FROM THE STANDARDIZED PATIENT

History

HPI: Mr. Green has had a bloody nose off and on for the past 3 months, always in the left nostril. Sometimes it just drips a little; some days it doesn't bleed at all. On two occasions it bled so much that Mr. Green thought he might have to call 9-1-1. The nosebleeds started with a bad cold at the beginning of winter. The cold resolved, but the nosebleeds are continuing. It is now February in Chicago, and the air has been dry in the house for the last 3 months. He has no pain.

The patient has been treating himself by pushing tissues up his nose. Sneezing and blowing his nose make it worse; nothing really seems to make it better. He has no nasal discharge (other than blood). He has had no trauma to the nose. He has also noticed that he has been bruising easily. He had never had problems with bleeding after dentistry. He has never had the current problem before. He sleeps through the night, unless it's a night when he wakes up with a nosebleed.

Allergies: Cats, dogs

Meds: Tylenol (15 tabs a day)

PMH: Other than for multiple knee surgeries from college football, the patient has never been hospitalized. He is still a little bitter that his college injuries kept him from playing for a professional team. He has no history of diabetes, hypertension, or heart disease.

The patient's last doctor informed him that he has premature osteoarthritis of the knees as a result of so many football injuries. He switched from aspirin to Tylenol when the nosebleed first began because he knows aspirin is a blood thinner. He denies any recent trauma or injuries.

He is on no special diet and usually eats junk food. He has had no problems urinating.

Family Hx: There is no family history of easy bruising.

Social Hx: He lives alone. He is currently out of work but has worked as a house painter in the past. He smokes a pack of cigarettes a day and admits that a friend brings over four 1-liter bottles of bourbon for him each Sunday, which lasts him the week. He admits to drinking in the morning but argues that that isn't why he's here. The patient denies using cocaine or recreational drugs.

Physical Exam

This patient's general appearance is slightly disheveled. He smells of alcohol and has some bloodstained tissue protruding from his left nares. His speech is slightly louder than usual, and he tries to give you a big hello and a slap on the back. His gait is slightly wobbly and his speech is a little slurred. His face appears yellow (yellow powder on skin). His sclera are clear. You will need to recognize that this is a jaundice case even though the patient will not be yellow all over.

Mr. Green's pupils are equal, round, and reactive to light. His extraocular movements are intact. His tympanic membranes are clear. There is no hemotympanum. His head is nontender to palpation. He removes the tissue from his right nostril upon your request, and your examination of the nose reveals no mass or active bleeding. The nose is nontender. There is no perforation in the septum. His neck is supple.

His lungs are clear to auscultation and his heart tones are regular. You may see that he has some palmar erythema (simulated by red powder on the hands) and spider angiomata on the skin (spidery marks drawn with a red pen). His abdomen is soft, with mild tenderness to the right upper quadrant. There is no pain under the right costal margin when the patient takes a deep breath. Liver span is normal to percussion. His extremities show some edema, and there are multiple old scars on his knees. He is alert to person, place, and time. He cannot remember three objects for a minute. He cannot spell the word *world* backward. He may appear defensive over your questions and refuse to answer them, exclaiming that he is "not in school anymore!" There is no facial asymmetry and his cranial nerves are intact. His motor strength is normal bilaterally. His gait is best described as wobbly.

THE CLOSING

By now you realize your patient is probably very intoxicated. This does not change how you act toward him. Show Mr. Green the same courtesy you show patients who are not intoxicated.

> **Doctor:** "Mr. Green, I have finished your physical exam. You told me you have had the bloody nose off and on for three months. You also have been using a lot of Tylenol and have been drinking about four liters of whiskey a week. On your exam I noticed that your skin is yellow and you are tender over the liver. The bloody noses are likely to be linked to a possible liver problem."

CHALLENGING QUESTIONS

Be prepared to answer the following type of challenging questions for this case:

> **Mr. Green:** "Are you saying you think I'm an alcoholic?"

> **Doctor:** "You are drinking a greater quantity of alcohol than what is recommended to stay healthy. I think we need to see if your liver is functioning normally or if the amount of alcohol you are drinking is damaging your liver."

SAMPLE PATIENT NOTE

History: Describe the history you just obtained from this patient. Include only information (pertinent positives and negatives) relevant to this patient's problem(s).

CC: Epistaxis

HPI: 3 mo of intermittent nosebleed. Sometimes heavy. Treated with tissue placed in the nose. It started after a URI. Always the L nares. Sneezing makes it worse, nothing makes it better. Denies trauma or discharge. Pt has noticed easy bruising lately. 1 gal whiskey a week. Last drink was right before he came to the clinic. No familial bleeding disorders.

Meds: Tylenol (15 tabs a day) for chronic knee pain. No aspirin or blood thinners.

PMH: No past history of nosebleeds or nasal surgery.
Hospitalizations—multiple orthopedic knee procedures in college.
+ osteoarthritis of knees. No DM/HTN. Heart disease.

FH: No familial bleeding disorders

SH: Lives alone, no cocaine or drug use, + smokes 2 ppd.

SAMPLE PATIENT NOTE

Physical Exam: Describe any positive and negative findings relevant to this patient's problem(s). Be careful to include *only* those parts of examination you performed in *this* encounter.

VS: 38.6°C, BP 110/80, HR 88, RR 18

GA: Pt smells of alcohol. Appears intoxicated and jaundiced. Palmar erythema, spider angiomata.

HEENT: PERRL EOMI. Nares—Bloody tissue in R nare. no active bleeding, no discharge tenderness or perforation of septum.
TM—clear, pharynx clear.

Abd: Soft, BS+, mild tenderness without rebound RUQ. Liver span NL to percussion.

Neuro: A + O × 3, memory poor, attention and concentration poor. FTN—bilateral dysmetria. Gait—ataxic.

Skin: Palmar erythema, spider angiomata, scattered bruises.

SAMPLE PATIENT NOTE

Data Interpretation: *Based on what you have learned from the history and physical examination,* list up to 3 diagnoses that might explain this patient's complaint(s). List your diagnoses from most to least likely. For some cases, fewer than 3 diagnoses will be appropriate. Then, enter the positive or negative findings from the history and the physical examination (if present) that support each diagnosis. Lastly, list initial *diagnostic* studies (if any) you would order for this patient (e.g., restricted physical exam maneuvers, laboratory tests, imaging, ECG, etc.).

Diagnosis #1: Epistaxis

Differential diagnosis and diagnostic reasoning

History Finding(s)	Physical Exam Finding(s)
Recurrent nosebleed	Blood in nose
Alcohol abuse	Jaundice
Acetaminophen ingestion—too high a dose	
Easy bruising	

Diagnosis #2: Liver insufficiency/failure

Differential diagnosis and diagnostic reasoning

History Finding(s)	Physical Exam Finding(s)
Alcohol abuse	Jaundice
Acetaminophen ingestion—too high a dose	Tender liver
	Easy bruising and bleeding, spider angiomata

Diagnosis #3: Alcohol intoxication

Differential diagnosis and diagnostic reasoning

History Finding(s)	Physical Exam Finding(s)
Admits to drinking last few hours	EtOH on breath
	Ataxia, dysmetria

Diagnostic Study/Studies

CBC, platelets

T. bili, AST, ALT, NH3

Acetaminophen level, EtOH

INR, lytes, glucose

Ultrasound RUQ

CASE DISCUSSION

Notes about the History-Taking

This case is a test of your ability to remain calm, cool, and professional during the challenges of dealing with a difficult patient. Mr. Green is obviously alcohol-intoxicated now, and he even curses during the encounter.

Be sure to ask how much Tylenol he is taking. Only if you ask why he takes Tylenol and how much he takes will you learn that he's taking about 5 grams of acetaminophen a day.

This case is complex because you need to delve deeper into the situation than just looking at the patient's nose. Examining the underlying problems of liver failure caused by a toxic combination of alcohol and Tylenol is the key to the case.

Notes about the Physical Exam

In alcoholic patients, always suspect head trauma, even if patients don't present with any complaints of trauma or head pain. Looking in the ears for hemotympanum provides valuable information because bleeding can sometimes be found with basilar skull fracture. Looking at the nose for possible trauma or lesions is important. As with all patients with a history of alcohol or drug use, be sure to do a mental status exam. Be sure to tell the patient about the simulated findings you see (the yellow makeup for jaundice and the red marks for spider angiomata).

Comments about the Patient Note

In addition to the differential diagnoses listed, hypoglycemia may also be present in this patient; it is common in alcoholics with poor liver function.

Case 7: **Sudden Abdominal Pain and Syncope**

DOORWAY INFORMATION

Opening Scenario

Sharon Hall is a 24 y/o female with sudden abdominal pain and syncope 20 minutes ago.

Vital Signs

- Temp: 37.0°C (98.6°F)
- BP: 90/65 mm Hg
- HR: 120/min
- RR: 24/min

Examinee Tasks

1. Obtain a focused history.
2. Perform a relevant physical examination. Do not perform rectal, pelvic, genitourinary, inguinal hernia, female breast, or corneal reflex examinations.
3. Discuss your initial diagnostic impression and your workup plan with the patient.
4. After leaving the room, complete your patient note on the given form.

BEFORE ENTERING THE ROOM

Clinical Reasoning: You will have noticed that this patient has *three abnormal vital signs*. Whatever has caused her to faint is still an active problem. In cases like this on the Step 2 CS, where the SP is portraying a very ill person with a life-threatening illness, you will need to pay very close attention to the doorway vital signs. Despite alarming vital signs, you will need to maintain a calm and reassuring tone throughout the encounter.

Ms. Hall is hypotensive, has a narrow pulse pressure, and is tachycardic and tachypneic. Hypovolemia is certainly a possibility. Think of causes of hypovolemia and abdominal pain in a young woman and you will have the correct diagnosis.

FROM THE STANDARDIZED PATIENT

History

HPI: The patient states she has had LLQ pain for the last week, with some lower abdominal/pelvic cramping, and about 3 hours ago it got much worse. The pain is now 6/10 intensity, and pain intensity has not changed in the last 3 hours. It feels very hot and sharp and is continuous. It radiates up to her left shoulder. She thought going to the bathroom would make it better. Urinating and defecating did not help. She looked, and there was no blood in the toilet. She stood up from the toilet and felt very dizzy, with no power to stand up. She is pretty sure she fainted completely. She woke up on the floor, kind of sweaty. She denies any injury from the fall. At that point her boyfriend drove her to see you at the hospital. She reports that for the last week she also had some vaginal discharge, more than her usual. She denies headache, shortness of breath, back pain, or dysuria. She feels nauseated. She denies vomiting or diarrhea. She has never had anything like this before. She has no history of trauma. She has been sleeping fine, with no special diet and no problems urinating.

Upon questioning about her menstrual cycle, Ms. Hall says she got her period 2 days ago. It is a little lighter than usual and 2 weeks later than her usual 28-day regular cycle. She is G0P0. Her only sexual partner is her new boyfriend and they do not consistently use contraception. They sometimes use condoms. She stopped taking the Pill a few months ago when she and her previous boyfriend broke up. She has never had a sexually transmitted disease.

Meds: Asthmacort, Ventolin inhaler, multivitamins

PMH: She was hospitalized 5 years ago for asthma attack. Her asthma is controlled with medications. She also had tubes put in her ears as a child for recurrent otitis.

Social Hx: Ms. Hall lives with her new boyfriend and her cat and works as a teacher's aide. She does not smoke, drink, or use recreational drugs.

Physical Exam

She looks a little pale and is sweaty. Her mental status is normal but she is slightly anxious from her abdominal pain. Pharynx is normal. Lungs are clear to auscultation. Ms. Hall's heart tones are rapid. Her abdomen appears normal. Bowel sounds are present. She has marked tenderness to light palpation in the left lower quadrant. She has rebound tenderness. No mass is appreciated. There is no CVA tenderness. She is alert. If asked to walk she gets dizzy and has a lot of pain.

THE CLOSING

Tell the patient in lay terms what might be wrong and which tests will provide the answer. Counsel her about any behaviors that impact her health. Finally, ask if she has any questions.

> **Doctor:** "Ms. Hall, I have finished your physical exam. Thanks for cooperating. I can see you are in a lot of pain. On your physical exam your heart rate is fast and you are very tender in your belly. I think this is most likely related to your period that is late. You could have a ruptured cyst. We'll need to do a pelvic exam, and I want you to have a pregnancy test and an ultrasound of your abdomen. Then we can know for sure what is causing the pain, and can plan treatment."

CHALLENGING QUESTIONS

Ms. Hall: "Am I pregnant?"

Doctor: "I'm concerned that with this much pain it could be a very abnormal pregnancy, a tubal pregnancy. Let me get this ultrasound for you quickly so we can find out."

SAMPLE PATIENT NOTE

History: Describe the history you just obtained from this patient. Include only information (pertinent positives and negatives) relevant to this patient's problem(s).

CC: Acute abdominal pain

HPI: Sudden onset 3 hrs ago, sharp/hot, 6/10 intensity LLQ pain. Pain is constant and radiates to L shoulder. Nothing makes it better. Standing up from toilet, had syncopal episode and was diaphoretic. LMP now, 2 weeks late and just spotting, lighter than usual. Periods usually regular with 3–5 pads on heaviest day. GOPO. Sexually active with new partner, no current birth control and unprotected sex. No previous episodes like this.
No vomiting, diarrhea, dysuria, or blood in urine or stool.

PMH: Asthma. Only one hospitalization for asthma, 5 years ago. No history of surgery. Meds—Ventolin, Azmacort inhalers.

SH: Lives with boyfriend. No smoking, EtOH, or drugs.

SAMPLE PATIENT NOTE

Physical Examination: Describe any positive and negative findings relevant to this patient's problem(s). Be careful to include only those parts of examination you performed in this encounter.

GA: In acute distress 2nd to pain, orthostatic on standing. BO 90/65, HR 120, RR 24, afebrile.

Chest: Clear to auscultation

Abd: Appears NL, scaphoid. BS+, very tender LLQ. No mass felt. + rebound LLQ. No CVA tenderness.

SAMPLE PATIENT NOTE

Data Interpretation: *Based on what you have learned from the history and physical examination,* list up to 3 diagnoses that might explain this patient's complaint(s). List your diagnoses from most to least likely. For some cases, fewer than 3 diagnoses will be appropriate. Then, enter the positive or negative findings from the history and the physical examination (if present) that support each diagnosis. Lastly, list initial *diagnostic* studies (if any) you would order for this patient (e.g., restricted physical exam maneuvers, laboratory tests, imaging, ECG, etc.).

Diagnosis #1: Ruptured ectopic pregnancy

Differential diagnosis and diagnostic reasoning

History Finding(s)	Physical Exam Finding(s)
Late period, then light bleeding	Orthostatic hypotension, tachycardia
Syncope	Diaphoretic
Abdominal pain that radiates to shoulder	+ rebound lower abdominal pain

Diagnosis #2: Pelvic inflammatory disease

Differential diagnosis and diagnostic reasoning

History Finding(s)	Physical Exam Finding(s)
Unprotected sex with new sexual partner	Abdominal pain
Vaginal discharge	

Diagnosis #3: Ruptured ovarian cyst

Differential diagnosis and diagnostic reasoning

History Finding(s)	Physical Exam Finding(s)
Syncope	Abdominal pain with peritoneal signs
Abdominal pain	
Radiates to shoulder	

Diagnostic Study/Studies

Complete pelvic and rectal exam

CBC

U/A, UCG, urine for GC/chlamydia

Quantitative HCG

Pelvic ultrasound

CASE DISCUSSION

Notes about the History-Taking

This patient is clearly at risk for either pregnancy (ectopic) or PID (pelvic inflammatory disease) given her symptoms and history of unprotected sex with a new sexual partner. A pelvic exam would likely move the differential in one direction or the other.

Notes about the Physical Exam

A complete abdominal exam consisting of inspection, observation, percussion, and palpation is warranted. You would not do deep palpation because there is already pain on light palpation, though you would still go ahead and check for peritonitis. The acceptable tests for peritonitis include: rebound tenderness, heel strike, bed shake, and percussing for tenderness. If the patient is tender to percussion, rebound doesn't need to be done.

Case 8: Vaginal Bleeding in a 40-Year-Old

DOORWAY INFORMATION

Opening Scenario

Carol Roberts is a 40 y/o woman who complains of "irregular vaginal bleeding."

Vital Signs

- Temp: 37.1°C (98.8°F)
- BP: 130/70 mm Hg
- HR: 100/min
- RR: 20/min
- BMI: 44

Examinee Tasks

1. Obtain a focused history.
2. Perform a relevant physical examination. Do not perform rectal, pelvic, genitourinary, inguinal hernia, female breast, or corneal reflex examinations.
3. Discuss your initial diagnostic impression and your workup plan with the patient.
4. After leaving the room, complete your patient note on the given form.

BEFORE ENTERING THE ROOM

Clinical Reasoning: Looking at the chief complaint, realize that a good Ob/Gyn and sexual history will be needed. You already know that a complete abdominal exam is indicated and that a pelvic exam will have to be ordered in the Diagnostic Studies.

The source of bleeding is usually uterine; only in the great minority of cases is the cervix or vagina going to be the source when there is bleeding in significant quantity. Pregnancy must always be excluded. Once it is, the classification for abnormal uterine bleeding in a reproductive-age woman is PALM-COEIN: **P**olyp, **A**denomyosis, **L**eiomyoma, **M**alignancy/hyperplasia, **C**oagulopathy, **O**vulatory dysfunction, **E**ndometrial, **I**atrogenic, **N**ot yet classified.

FROM THE STANDARDIZED PATIENT

History

HPI: Ms. Roberts complains of irregular and heavy periods in the last 6 months. She states she has only had maybe two normal periods in the last 6 months. Normally her period lasts 3 to 5 days, but it is now lasting 8 to 10 days. Having such long periods is making it harder to track her cycles. She is having to use pads in addition to super-size tampons. There is sometimes pain and/or cramps. She denies any fever or discharge. She states she is not having hot flashes.

Sometimes she gets a little irritable around her period, but not always. That has not changed in many years. She is just finishing her period for 10 days now. She made an appointment because she felt a little lightheaded when she stood up suddenly and ran for the bus yesterday. There was mild shortness of breath with running, though no chest pain, syncope, or palpitations. This is the first time she has experienced this. She reports a very significant permanent weight gain, 25 or 30 pounds, with her first pregnancy, and she gained more weight with the second pregnancy 18 years ago. She has had no problems urinating. She denies any excess hair on her body but says she does have to shave her chin.

Her previous period was 4 weeks ago and also long and heavy. She started have periods at age 12. Ms. Roberts has been pregnant twice; she had two children and had one abortion when she was 16. She has not been sexually active for two years. She has only been sexually active with men. Ms. Roberts is divorced and has two college-age children that usually live at school. She works as the day manager of a small retail business. She smokes one pack of cigarettes per day and drinks two drinks maybe once a week, when on a date. She does not use any recreational drugs.

PMH: She has been hospitalized for 2 cesarean sections only. Ms. Roberts denies diabetes mellitus, hypertension, and heart disease.

Allergies: Amoxicillin

Meds/vitamins: She has not used birth control pills in 5 years.

Physical Exam

The patient appears slightly pale. The SP may demonstrate that by having a little white makeup on her cheeks or forehead. In this way the SP can give you the simulated physical finding of pallor, indicating anemia.

Ms. Roberts is awake and alert. She is obese. Her thyroid is not enlarged. Heart tones are regular. Her abdomen appears normal. Bowel sounds are normal. There are no masses or tenderness, specifically in the suprapubic and lower quadrants on both sides. There is no costovertebral angle tenderness. There is no cyanosis or edema to the extremities. Her gait is normal.

THE CLOSING

There is a good chance that Ms. Roberts's problem may be related to her obesity. This issue needs to be handled carefully, since many patients are ashamed of their weight.

Doctor: "Ms. Roberts, I'm ready to tell you what I am thinking. First, I want to make sure I understand. For the last 6 months you have been having periods that are heavier than normal. And yesterday you got a little lightheaded and short of breath. I think you may be anemic from the heavy periods. That would explain all your symptoms and being pale too. In order to figure out why you're having so much bleeding, I'd like to order some blood tests and an ultrasound of your uterus."

CHALLENGING QUESTIONS

Ms. Roberts: "Do you think I could have cancer?"

Doctor: "It's not the most common cause of this problem, but with the ultrasound we will be able to tell if a biopsy of the lining of your uterus is necessary."

SAMPLE PATIENT NOTE

History: Describe the history you just obtained from this patient. Include only information (pertinent positives and negatives) relevant to this patient's problem(s).

CC: Vaginal bleeding

HPI: Periods were normal until last 6 months of irregular, sometimes painful heavy periods with heavier than usual blood loss needing pads in addition to tampons. Periods can last 10 days. No fever, chills, dysuria, abdominal pain, or discharge. + dyspnea with exertion and some lightheadedness when stands up fast. Has never had irregular periods before. LMP ending now, started 10 days ago. Menarche age 12. Not sexually active for last 2 years. Gained 25–30 pounds with pregnancies.

PMH: Hospitalized for two C-sections. No trauma or other surg.
        Denies DM, HTN, heart disease.
        Meds—vitamins, not on hormones for past 5 years.

ROS: No change in her sleep pattern.
        + dieting 1,200 cals/day. Not a vegetarian.

SH: Lives alone, states well adjusted to kids being in school. Smokes 1 ppd, EtoH 2 drinks "on a date." No recreational drugs.

SAMPLE PATIENT NOTE

Physical Examination: Describe any positive and negative findings relevant to this patient's problem(s). Be careful to include *only* those parts of examination you performed in *this* encounter.

VS: T 98.8°F, BP 130/70, HR 100, RR 20

GA: Looks pale, NAD, obese

CVS: S1 S2 NL, no GRM

Abd: Appears NL, BS+, no masses or tenderness all 4 Q, no suprapubic pain, no CVA pain

SAMPLE PATIENT NOTE

Data Interpretation: *Based on what you have learned from the history and physical examination,* list up to 3 diagnoses that might explain this patient's complaint(s). List your diagnoses from most to least likely. For some cases, fewer than 3 diagnoses will be appropriate. Then, enter the positive or negative findings from the history and the physical examination (if present) that support each diagnosis. Lastly, list initial *diagnostic* studies (if any) you would order for this patient (e.g., restricted physical exam maneuvers, laboratory tests, imaging, ECG, etc.).

Diagnosis #1: Leiomyoma (fibroids)

Differential diagnosis and diagnostic reasoning

History Finding(s)	Physical Exam Finding(s)
Heavy periods past 6 months	Looks pale
Increased abdominal cramping with menses	Tachycardia

Diagnosis #2: Polycystic ovarian syndrome (PCOS)

Differential diagnosis and diagnostic reasoning

History Finding(s)	Physical Exam Finding(s)
Irregular menses	Obesity
Hirsutism	

Diagnosis #3: Endometrial hyperplasia, r/o endometrial cancer

Differential diagnosis and diagnostic reasoning

History Finding(s)	Physical Exam Finding(s)
Heavy, irregular menses	

Diagnostic Study/Studies

Complete pelvic exam

CBC, DHEA-S, testosterone

Pelvic ultrasound

CASE DISCUSSION

Notes about the History-Taking

In this case, the gynecological history is of prime importance. Determining risk for pregnancy allows you to proceed with a differential in a nonpregnant woman.

Notes about the Physical Exam

Certainly some heart and lung exams are indicated because the patient was a little short of breath with exertion due to the anemia. Also, the chief complaint of vaginal bleeding indicates that a fairly complete abdominal exam is going to be on the checklist as well.

Comments about the Patient Note

Since there are many possible diagnoses for dysfunctional uterine bleeding, it is important to look for signs and symptoms that point you toward either structural diagnoses (uterine fibroids) or hormonal diagnoses (PCOS). Know the most common diagnoses, but don't miss other diagnoses (endometrial cancer).

Case 9: **Fever and Weight Loss**

BEFORE ENTERING THE ROOM

Clinical Reasoning: This patient has three abnormal vital signs (temperature, heart rate, and respiratory rate).

When two symptoms are given in the opening scenario, it is likely that the final diagnosis will explain both symptoms. It is much less likely that the patient will have two completely unrelated problems. Because weight loss takes some time to notice, this situation is probably not an acute febrile illness; it is more likely to be something chronic or subacute. Patient's vital signs indicate that he is tachypneic. Remember that in addition to pulmonary and cardiac causes, metabolic acidosis is also a potential cause of tachypnea.

FROM THE STANDARDIZED PATIENT

History

HPI: Mr. Brown comes to you and tells you he has been sick for most of the past month. It started at that time with fever, headache, malaise, and swollen glands. That lasted about 3 months. He went to a different clinic and a mono test was done, but that turned out negative. Then he started to get fevers, cough, and shortness of breath with exertion. The SOB is only with exercise. He has stopped exercising completely. The fever is now intermittent.

The cough is nonproductive. There is occasionally some mild chest discomfort with coughing. Nothing seems to make it better or worse. He has been sleeping more than usual lately and often wakes up at night with soaked clothing and sheets. He has lost approximately 20 lb. and has a decreased appetite. He has no problem urinating. He is sexually active, with 4 different sexual partners in the last year, 3 female and 1 male. He has not consistently practiced safe sex. To his knowledge none of his past sexual partners is ill. He had a negative HIV test 3 years ago.

Prior to this past month, Mr. Brown was perfectly healthy. He is upset that he has been missing so much work due to illness recently. He denies a travel history. He denies any known exposure to tuberculosis but doesn't remember ever having a PPD.

Allergies: None

Meds: Tylenol and Motrin for fever, without relief

PMH: Mr. Brown has never been hospitalized. He has had not surgery or trauma. He denies diabetes, hypertension, and heart disease.

Social Hx: Mr. Brown lives alone. He is a social worker for the state child protective agency. He does not smoke, drink, or use any recreational drugs.

Physical Exam

Mr. Brown looks unhappy. He is 145 lb and is 5 feet 9 inches. Occasionally during the interview he has a dry, hacking cough.

His neck is supple. Lungs are clear to auscultation. Tactile fremitus, percussion, and auscultation are normal. His heart tones are fast without any murmur or gallop. When you check for cervical and supraclavicular adenopathy, he tells you that his glands feel swollen and tender. His abdomen is soft and nontender. Bowel sounds are normal. Gait is normal. He is alert and does not seem confused.

THE CLOSING

Doctor: "It is hard to know for sure what is causing your symptoms, but we need to start by ruling out some possible causes of infection."

Mr. Brown: "Do you think I might have AIDS?"

Doctor: "Yes, it could be. But you need to have a blood test to be sure. I would also like to take a picture of your chest to look for pneumonia as well. Since you've never had a PPD test, we will also check for tuberculosis, or TB."

Mr. Brown: "Am I dying?"

Doctor: "What you have might be serious, but whatever we find, I'll be able to provide you with good treatment. I am very glad you came to see me today."

SAMPLE PATIENT NOTE

History: Describe the history you just obtained from this patient. Include only information (pertinent positives and negatives) relevant to this patient's problem(s).

CC: Cough, fever, wt loss

HPI: 10-lb. weight loss in last month. Illness began with fever, fatigue, diffuse adenopathy, and night sweats. Now has nonproductive cough, SOB, DOE, and intermittent fevers. Pt has been missing a lot of work. Nothing seems to make it better or worse. No known HIV or TB contacts. Multiple sexual partners, 1 male partner, unprotected sex. Denies IVDU. No syncope or confusion.

Allergies: None

Meds: Tylenol and Motrin for fever

PMH: Never hospitalized. No trauma or surgery. No TB, DM.

ROS: No diarrhea

SH: Lives alone, works as social worker. No smoking, alcohol, IV, or rec drugs.

SAMPLE PATIENT NOTE

Physical Examination: Describe any positive and negative findings relevant to this patient's problem(s). Be careful to include *only* those parts of examination you performed in *this* encounter.

VS: Temp: 100.8°F, HR: 110, RR: 24, BP: 110/80

GA: Looks chronically ill

HEENT: Pharynx clear. Neck supple. Tender over cervical nodes, no supraclavicular adenopathy.

Axilla: No adenopathy.

Chest: Clear to A + P. Normal fremitus.

CV: Tachycardic. No obvious murmur, rub, or gallop.

Abd: Soft, nontender

SAMPLE PATIENT NOTE

Data Interpretation: *Based on what you have learned from the history and physical examination,* list up to 3 diagnoses that might explain this patient's complaint(s). List your diagnoses from most to least likely. For some cases, fewer than 3 diagnoses will be appropriate. Then, enter the positive or negative findings from the history and the physical examination (if present) that support each diagnosis. Lastly, list initial *diagnostic* studies (if any) you would order for this patient (e.g., restricted physical exam maneuvers, laboratory tests, imaging, ECG, etc.).

Diagnosis #1: Acute retroviral syndrome (HIV seroconversion)

Differential diagnosis and diagnostic reasoning

History Finding(s)	**Physical Exam Finding(s)**
Multiple sex partners of both genders, does not practice safe sex	Looks ill
+ 10 pound weight loss, fevers	Tenderness over lymph nodes
Diffuse adenopathy	
Fatigue, night sweats	

Diagnosis #2: Tuberculosis

Differential diagnosis and diagnostic reasoning

History Finding(s)	**Physical Exam Finding(s)**
Fever, cough, weight loss, night sweats for several weeks	Tenderness over lymph nodes
Shortness of breath	

Diagnosis #3: Hodgkin's lymphoma

Differential diagnosis and diagnostic reasoning

History Finding(s)	**Physical Exam Finding(s)**
Pt has B symptoms of weight loss, fevers, and night sweats	Tenderness over lymph nodes

Diagnostic Study/Studies

CXR, measure O_2% (pulse Ox), CBC

CD4, PPD, quantiferon

CASE DISCUSSION

Notes about the Physical Exam

The sicker the case the SP is portraying, the harder it is to visualize. This patient is giving you historical symptoms strongly suggestive of potential pulmonary infection. However, the actor is not going to be able to simulate abnormal breath sounds. He probably will cough a couple of times during the exam to remind you he really has pneumonia-like signs and symptoms. While the SP won't have enlarged lymph nodes, you can interpret the tenderness observed during palpation over the lymph nodes as a finding of adenopathy.

Comments about the Patient Note

The differential here is potentially broad. Always think in terms of the best initial tests that will help narrow the differential and direct further care. Do not worry about tests the patient may need later in his illness.

Case 10: **Adolescent Weight Loss**

DOORWAY INFORMATION

Opening Scenario

Amy Wright is a 17 y/o female who comes to the clinic brought in by her grandmother, who is concerned that Amy is losing weight.

Vital Signs

- Temp: 36.3°C (97.4°F)
- BP: 85/50 mm Hg
- HR: 60/min, regular
- RR: 14/min

Examinee Tasks

1. Obtain a focused history.
2. You will not be required to perform a physical examination in this case.
3. Discuss your initial diagnostic impression and your workup plan with the patient.
4. After leaving the room, complete your patient note on the given form.

BEFORE ENTERING THE ROOM

Clinical Reasoning: Causes of weight loss can include the following:

- Depression
- Anorexia nervosa
- Hyperthyroidism
- Drug use
- Cancer
- Diabetes

Note the abnormal vital signs. When an adolescent is brought in by a worried family member, you may need to work on forming an alliance with the adolescent and assure them of confidentiality.

FROM THE PATIENT

History

HPI: Amy lets you know that she is here because her grandmother is worried about her losing weight but that she feels just fine. Amy lives with her grandmother because her mother died a year and a half ago after being hit by a drunk driver. Amy is a gymnast in high school and has a goal of being on the Olympic team. She says her coach wants her to keep her weight down. She thinks she has recovered from the death of her mother, but her grandmother is constantly hovering over her and trying to get her to eat. Amy has lost about 20 lb. in the last 6 months. She is 5 feet 3 inches, and 105 lb. She says she has cut out all desserts and is trying to eat healthy. She denies vomiting. Amy is very concerned about her weight and looks, and feels she is still too heavy to make the Olympic team. She realizes she must be strong also. Amy's frustration with her weight makes it hard to enjoy gymnastics sometimes. Amy complains of frequently feeling hot, as well as being sweaty a lot of the time. She drinks a lot of ice water to "cleanse her system."

Amy does seem to urinate frequently; however, she has no burning or pain with urination. She is sleeping less than usual, now about 6 hours a night. She claims to be up late doing homework. She has no constipation or diarrhea. She has two bowel movements a day. Amy is not sure when her last period was. She is not sexually active. Amy states she does not smoke or use alcohol or drugs.

She still has periods of sadness over her mother's death 18 months ago. She has not been in contact with her friends outside of gymnastics. Her grades are slipping a little. Amy says classes are boring and she can't concentrate. She denies ever being so sad that she has wanted to kill herself.

Amy takes no medicine other than a multivitamin, and she has no allergies.

PMH: Amy has never been hospitalized and has had no surgery or trauma. She has never had any major illnesses.

Family Hx: Amy does not know what happened to her father, who left 14 years ago. Her mother was healthy before the accident.

Physical Exam

There is no physical exam in this case.

THE CLOSING

It will be important to get Amy's permission to share your thoughts with Amy's grandmother.

> **Doctor:** "Amy, I'm concerned that you are losing a lot of weight and are very thin but think that you are overweight. I'm also concerned about how sad you seem and wonder if it's been really hard to cope with losing your mother. I'd like to do a physical exam and some blood tests to see if there are any physical problems that have resulted from or could be causing your weight loss."

SAMPLE PATIENT NOTE

History: Describe the history you just obtained from this patient. Include only information (pertinent positives and negatives) relevant to this patient's problem(s).

CC: *Weight loss*

HPI: *20-lb. weight loss in the last 6 mo. Now 5'3", 105 lb. Poor appetite. States wants to keep weight down for gymnastics team. She denies vomiting. Amy lives with grandparents after death of mother 18 mo ago. No alcohol, cigarettes, or recreational drugs. Poor body image, thinks she is still too heavy to make Olympic team. Does not seem to be enjoying gymnastics anymore, frequently sad. Has few friends, grades are dropping, and cannot concentrate. No known suicidal ideation. Pt sleeping less than usual, about 6 hrs/night. Frequently feels hot, is frequently thirsty, and drinks a lot of ice water.*

      LMP—unsure; irregular menses. Not sexually active.

      NKMA; Meds: Multivitamin

PMH: *No hospitalizations, trauma, major illness, or surgery*

ROS: *No dysuria, hematuria. No constipation or diarrhea. Has 2 bowel movements/day.*

FH: *Amy's mother was healthy prior to her fatal car accident. No known hx for father. No family history of depression.*

SAMPLE PATIENT NOTE

Physical Examination: Describe any positive and negative findings relevant to this patient's problem(s). Be careful to include *only* those parts of examination you performed in *this* encounter.

There is no physical exam in this case.

SAMPLE PATIENT NOTE

Data Interpretation: *Based on what you have learned from the history and physical examination,* list up to 3 diagnoses that might explain this patient's complaint(s). List your diagnoses from most to least likely. For some cases, fewer than 3 diagnoses will be appropriate. Then, enter the positive or negative findings from the history and the physical examination (if present) that support each diagnosis. Lastly, list initial *diagnostic* studies (if any) you would order for this patient (e.g., restricted physical exam maneuvers, laboratory tests, imaging, ECG, etc.).

Diagnosis #1: Anorexia nervosa

Differential diagnosis and diagnostic reasoning

History Finding(s)	Physical Exam Finding(s)
Poor body image—pt thinks she is too fat	
20 lb. weight loss, irregular menses	
Involved in gymnastics, where there is an emphasis on weight	

Diagnosis #2: Depression

Differential diagnosis and diagnostic reasoning

History Finding(s)	Physical Exam Finding(s)
Death of parent	
Reported as sad, can't concentrate, decreasing grades	
Loss of enjoyment of activity (gymnastics), poor appetite, sleep disturbance	

Diagnosis #3: Hyperthyroidism

Differential diagnosis and diagnostic reasoning

History Finding(s)	Physical Exam Finding(s)
Unexplained 20 lb. weight loss	
Frequently feels hot, drinking ice water, disrupted sleep	

Diagnostic Study/Studies

Physical exam

TSH, T4, FT4

CBC, lytes, BUN, Cr, Glu

U/A, UCG

CASE DISCUSSION

With a chief complaint of weight loss, be sure to ask if the weight loss is intentional and assess dietary habits and exercise. Weight loss is most commonly simply a result of eating less, exercising more, or some combination of the two. The differential of weight loss in the absence of this then leads to other metabolic derangements such as hyperthyroidism, diabetes, or (less commonly) malignancy. Even if the cause of symptoms seems to be psychological, it is always correct to broaden your search for medical illnesses that might be causing psychiatric symptoms.

Notes about the History-Taking

With an adolescent history, in a nonacute clinical encounter, remember to ask about the following history items:

- Home: Good relationship with grandmother
- Education: Doing less well in school
- Activities: Enjoying gymnastics less
- Drugs: Denies
- Sex: Not sexually active
- Suicide/depression: Frequently sad, not enjoying gymnastics. No suicidal ideation.

Case 11: **Bed-Wetting in a 7-Year-Old Child**

DOORWAY INFORMATION

Opening Scenario

Mrs. Susan Jackson comes to speak with you about her son, Jason, who is 7 years old and still wets the bed.

Vital Signs

N/A

Examinee Tasks

1. Obtain a focused history.
2. You will not be required to perform a physical examination in this case.
3. Discuss your initial diagnostic impression and your workup plan with the patient.
4. After leaving the room, complete your patient note on the given form.

BEFORE ENTERING THE ROOM

Clinical Reasoning: It is important to distinguish secondary bed-wetting in a child who previously stayed dry at night to primary bed-wetting in children who have always struggled with this problem.

Enuresis is a very common complaint in children. It is often hereditary and not due to any medical or psychiatric illness, and most cases resolve spontaneously. As with any symptom, it is important to obtain the intensity, onset, and quantity, as well as any factors that make it better or worse. Ask about any recent stressors. When discussing associated symptoms, ask questions to assess for possible constipation, UTI, or diabetes mellitus, as these are common causes of secondary enuresis.

While taking the past medical history, specifically ask about how the bed-wetting is affecting the child's self-esteem. Determine the parents' reaction to the bed-wetting, since emotional trauma inflicted by the parent(s) may be a larger problem than the dirty laundry. In place of the physical exam, a pediatric history will need to be completed. Counseling and teaching parents about enuresis during the closing will be a prominent component of this case.

FROM THE GUARDIAN

History

HPI: Mrs. Jackson states that her son, Jason, has always been a bed-wetter. It occurred in early childhood, when he was never able to reliably stay dry through the night. It was much better from age 5.5 to 7 but now has started to happen again frequently since his father was redeployed to Afghanistan. Bed-wetting happens about once a week. It seems to happen more frequently when he stays with his grandparents. It is a bigger problem when he wets the bed at the grandparents' home because they criticize Jason about it. Mrs. Jackson has come to accept it and just knows she will frequently need to wash the sheets. The mattress is protected with a plastic cover that can be wiped down. Unfortunately, Mrs. Jackson has to travel on business frequently and the bed-wetting has become more of a source of conflict lately between the grandparents and grandchild. Not drinking fluids before bed sometimes prevents bed-wetting—but having a lot of liquids prior to bed doesn't always lead to bed-wetting. The Jacksons have tried having Jason urinate right before bed, and even setting the alarm clock for 2 A.M. so he can go to the bathroom. He has no dysuria, weight loss, or polydipsia. He has never fainted. He has a bowel movement every 3 or 4 days, and sometimes he has to strain to move his bowels.

Ped Hx: Mrs. Jackson tells you she received regular prenatal care during her pregnancy. She did not smoke or use drugs or alcohol. Jason was a full-term baby and delivered vaginally. Jason weighed 7 lb 6 oz and was 21 inches at birth. He had no problems with jaundice, breathing, or eating, and she recalls they went home within 24 hours after his birth.

Jason's father, who is currently deployed in Afghanistan, had a history of bed-wetting until he was 11 years old. There is increased stress at home worrying about Mr. Jackson. The grandparents never hit, scream at, or act neglectfully toward Jason, but Mrs. Jackson is aware of how their remarks about bed-wetting affect him.

PMH: Jason takes no prescription medications and has no allergies. He has never been hospitalized or had any surgery or trauma. His sleep pattern is normal and he does not snore. He sometimes complains of constipation or abdominal pain.

Jason was breast-fed and was weaned at age 8 months to milk and solid food. He now takes a pediatric vitamin every day and Mrs. Jackson states she tries to put nutritious food on the table. He eats a lot of cheese and frequently needs to strain when defecating. Jason started walking at age 1 year, and was toilet-trained by age 2.5 years (except for this bed-wetting problem). His immunizations are up to date. He gets regular pediatric checkups.

Physical Exam

There is no physical exam in this case.

THE CLOSING

Doctor: "Well, as it sounds like you know, most cases of bed-wetting are just normal and the child eventually outgrows them. But you are concerned about his grandparents' comments and their effect on Jason. I would be happy to call your parents and speak with them if you think it will help. I also want to see Jason for a physical exam, and I will check his urine. Right now, the other thing is to suggest that Jason eat more vegetables and fruit and a little less cheese. Sometimes constipation can make this problem worse. Do you have any questions for me?"

CHALLENGING QUESTIONS

Mrs. Jackson: "I've read there are some medicines that prevent bed-wetting. Can you give me a prescription?"

Doctor: "I need to examine Jason and collect a urine sample to make sure there are no medical problems causing the bed-wetting. Usually, bed-wetting is just a normal developmental stage. It is very hereditary, so your husband's history makes this likely."

SAMPLE PATIENT NOTE

History: Describe the history you just obtained from this patient. Include only information (pertinent positives and negatives) relevant to this patient's problem(s).

CC: *7 y/o son with enuresis*

HPI: *Bed-wetting in child who was toilet-trained at age 2.5 yrs. Improved greatly from age 5.5 to 7, now wets bed about once a week. Symptoms started again when father sent to Afghanistan. Mother states grandparents sometimes "belittle" the child regarding enuresis. Mother has no other concerns regarding grandparents' care of child. Nothing reliably makes it better or worse. No dysuria, polyuria, or polydipsia. No fever. Has bowel movement every 3–4 days. Sometimes constipated.*

     Allergies: None

     Meds: Pediatric vitamins

PMH: *No hospitalizations, trauma, or surgery*

ROS: *Sleeps 9 hours a night, no snoring. No weight loss. Eats a lot of cheese. Has bowel movement q 3–4 d.*

FH: *Father wet bed until age 11*

Ped Hx: *Full-term vaginal delivery. + Prenatal care. No drugs or alcohol. No complications in neonatal period. Toilet-trained at 2.5 yrs and walked at 12 months.*

SAMPLE PATIENT NOTE

Physical Examination: Describe any positive and negative findings relevant to this patient's problem(s). Be careful to include *only* those parts of examination you performed in *this* encounter.

There is no physical exam in this case.

SAMPLE PATIENT NOTE

Data Interpretation: *Based on what you have learned from the history and physical examination*, list up to 3 diagnoses that might explain this patient's complaint(s). List your diagnoses from most to least likely. For some cases, fewer than 3 diagnoses will be appropriate. Then, enter the positive or negative findings from the history and the physical examination (if present) that support each diagnosis. Lastly, list initial *diagnostic* studies (if any) you would order for this patient (e.g., restricted physical exam maneuvers, laboratory tests, imaging, ECG, etc.).

Diagnosis #1: Primary nocturnal enuresis

Differential diagnosis and diagnostic reasoning

History Finding(s)	Physical Exam Finding(s)
Patient with bed-wetting since toilet trained	
Father with enuresis until age 11	

Diagnosis #2: Secondary enuresis from constipation

Differential diagnosis and diagnostic reasoning

History Finding(s)	Physical Exam Finding(s)
Constipation	
Enuresis got better, then was worse	

Diagnosis #3: Adjustment disorder

Differential diagnosis and diagnostic reasoning

History Finding(s)	Physical Exam Finding(s)
Enuresis was better until father left for military deployment	
Mother travels frequently leaving child with grandparents	

Diagnostic Study/Studies

Schedule child for physical exam

Blood glucose, urinalysis

CASE DISCUSSION

Notes about the History-Taking

All enuresis cases require a family history because primary nocturnal enuresis is genetic. Always ask about dietary history, since constipation is another cause of enuresis. Cystitis is also a common cause of enuresis, so be sure to ask about symptoms of a urinary tract infection. In this case, enuresis has been persistent rather than secondary or new-onset, making cystitis much less likely.

Psychological stress may also be a cause in this case, and is more likely since the child's bed-wetting got worse only after his father was deployed. It is important to take the social history, and also to understand the parents' and other caregivers' response to bed-wetting.

Comments about the Patient Note

A physical exam and U/A are required on all cases of enuresis.

Case 12: Right Upper Quadrant Abdominal Pain

DOORWAY INFORMATION

Opening Scenario

Larry Mitchell is a 52 y/o male who comes to the clinic complaining of RUQ pain.

Vital Signs

- Temp: 37.0°C (98.6°F)
- BP: 160/90 mm Hg
- HR: 90/min
- RR 16/min

Examinee Tasks

1. Obtain a focused history.
2. Perform a relevant physical examination. Do not perform rectal, pelvic, genitourinary, inguinal hernia, female breast, or corneal reflex examinations.
3. Discuss your initial diagnostic impression and your workup plan with the patient.
4. After leaving the room, complete your patient note on the given form.

BEFORE ENTERING THE ROOM

Clinical Reasoning: For any case of abdominal pain, location can immediately help you to start a differential by thinking anatomically of what organs can cause pain in that area or quadrant. Then match patient's risk factors and symptom complex to the most likely diagnosis.

FROM THE STANDARDIZED PATIENT

History

HPI: Mr. Mitchell came to the clinic because he felt he should "get checked out." He occasionally gets pain in his upper abdomen and at times underneath the right rib cage. He last had the upper abdominal pain for most of the night after a pepperoni pizza for dinner 2 nights ago, but now the pain is now gone. The pain can be from 1/10 to 4/10 and lasts anywhere from a few minutes to a few hours. It feels like a "hot" pain, and it started about 3 months ago. Now the pain occurs a few times a week and seems to be getting worse in intensity and duration. It sometimes moves to his back just at the right shoulder blade. He notices it more after eating fatty foods.

The pain does not get worse when he walks. Bending over exacerbates the pain. There has been no black or red bowel movement and no other change in his bowel movement pattern. Patient has never experienced this before. It seems better when he takes some acetaminophen or ibuprofen. He tried Mylanta without any relief. Has 2 beers almost every night during the week and scotch on the weekend. He gets annoyed at those who criticize his drinking and does not feel guilty. He doesn't drink in the morning. He has tried to cut back on occasion when he's dieting and trying to lose weight.

He has no chest pain, SOB, vomiting, diarrhea, dysuria, or rash. He has not had any change in his sleep pattern, his weight has been slowly increasing each year, and he has no problem urinating.

He takes no medicine regularly and has no allergies.

PMH: He was hospitalized once for appendicitis 35 years ago. He has had no trauma or other surgery. He denies any history of DM, HTN, or heart disease.

Family Hx: Patient's parents both smoked heavily and died in their early 70s from heart disease and cancer, respectively.

Social Hx: He is sexually active when he has a girlfriend. He is single at the moment. He is divorced and sells cars for a living. He stopped smoking 20 years ago. Never used recreational drugs.

Physical Exam

Mr. Mitchell is 6 feet 2 inches and 240 lb. He is in no distress. He last had the upper abdominal pain for most of the night after a pepperoni pizza for dinner 2 nights ago, but now the pain is now gone. His skin has normal color and there is no makeup on him to indicate that he is jaundiced. His pharynx is clear. Carotid upstrokes are normal without bruits. His lungs are clear. There is no jugular venous distention. Heart tones are normal. Abdomen is obese. He had mild epigastric tenderness. There is no rebound. Murphy's sign is negative.

The patient is alert. There is no pain when the RUQ is palpated and the patient inhales. His bowel sounds are normal and there is normal tympany to all four quadrants with percussion. There is no back tenderness. Extremities reveal no edema.

THE CLOSING

Doctor: "Mr. Mitchell, I'd like to tell you what I am thinking. I think this pain in your belly might be from acid in the stomach or due to alcohol. I'd like you to have blood tests today to find out the cause. I'm also concerned that your blood pressure is high, which also might be due to the amount of alcohol you drink. What's your thinking about your alcohol intake?"

CHALLENGING QUESTIONS

Following is an example of how you should counsel patients about weight loss.

Mr. Mitchell: "I find it difficult to lose weight and have tried different diets over the years. Is there something else I can do?"

Doctor: "Yes, I know that it can be difficult to lose weight. Increasing fruits and vegetables in your diet and being more active is an important first step. Also, be careful to avoid high-fat and high-sugar foods. I'll have you speak with our nutrition expert, who can help to plan out a diet and exercise program with you."

SAMPLE PATIENT NOTE

History: Describe the history you just obtained from this patient. Include only information (pertinent positives and negatives) relevant to this patient's problem(s).

CC: Abdominal pain

HPI: Epigastric and RUQ pain. 1/10 increasing to 4/10 pain described as hot. Started 3 mo ago, getting more frequent, and lasting longer. No pain now. Pain all night after pizza. Significant alcohol intake: CAGE 2/4 and at-risk drinking.

Made worse by fatty foods and sometimes when bends over. Better with acetaminophen and ibuprofen, no relief with Mylanta. No SOB, chest pain, nausea, vomiting, diarrhea, dysuria, or rash. No blood in stool.

Medications: No regular medications

PMH: Appendectomy 35 yrs ago. No trauma, no h/o DM, HTN, heart disease.

ROS: Slowly gaining weight over years. No change in sleep pattern, no problem urinating.

FH: Parents died from heart disease and cancer

SH: Divorced, lives alone, works as car salesman. Stopped smoking 20 years ago. No drugs.

SAMPLE PATIENT NOTE

Physical Examination: Describe any positive and negative findings relevant to this patient's problem(s). Be careful to include *only* those parts of examination you performed in *this* encounter.

VS: 98.6 160/90 90 16 obese

GA: NAD. 6'2", 240 lb.

HEENT: Sclera NL, palate without jaundice. No JVD.

Abd: Appears NL; BS+, + moderate RUQ tenderness to palpation. NL percussion. Neg Murphy's.

SAMPLE PATIENT NOTE

Data Interpretation: *Based on what you have learned from the history and physical examination,* list up to 3 diagnoses that might explain this patient's complaint(s). List your diagnoses from most to least likely. For some cases, fewer than 3 diagnoses will be appropriate. Then, enter the positive or negative findings from the history and the physical examination (if present) that support each diagnosis. Lastly, list initial *diagnostic* studies (if any) you would order for this patient (e.g., restricted physical exam maneuvers, laboratory tests, imaging, ECG, etc.).

Diagnosis #1: Gastroesophageal reflux disease

Differential diagnosis and diagnostic reasoning

History Finding(s)	Physical Exam Finding(s)
Weight gain	Tender epigastrium
Epigastric pain after eating	No fever
Worse with bending over	No jaundice

Diagnosis #2: Pancreatitis

Differential diagnosis and diagnostic reasoning

History Finding(s)	Physical Exam Finding(s)
Epigastric pain	Tender epigastric region
Drinks 2/day	

Diagnosis #3: Biliary colic/gallstone

Differential diagnosis and diagnostic reasoning

History Finding(s)	Physical Exam Finding(s)
RUQ pain after fatty foods	Tender epigastric area

Diagnostic Study/Studies

Rectal with FOBT

T. bili, AST, ALT, alk phos

Ultrasound of gallbladder

Upper endoscopy

Amylase, lipase

CASE DISCUSSION

Comments about the Patient Note

This man has a series of various symptoms that may have a series of different causes when you first elicit the history. You should think to yourself, are they related to the gastrointestinal system—gallbladder, pancreatitis, gastrointestinal ulcer? These are all possibilities.

Your workup plan will help to determine the likely diagnosis based on the information you have found. Remember to include the most common and most likely differential diagnoses and avoid including obscure or unusual conditions.

Case 13: **Mental Status Changes**

DOORWAY INFORMATION

Opening Scenario

David Miller Sr. is a 90 y/o male who is here for medication refills.

Vital Signs

- Temp: 37.0°C (98.2°F)
- BP: 165/85 mm Hg
- HR: 85/min
- RR 18/min

Examinee Tasks

1. Obtain a focused history.
2. Discuss your initial diagnostic impression and your workup plan with the patient.
3. After leaving the room, complete your patient note on the given form.

BEFORE ENTERING THE ROOM

Clinical Reasoning: Based on the Doorway Information, you can anticipate that this case involves an elderly patient who might require mental status evaluation. Functional assessment activities of daily living (ADLs) and instrumental activities of daily living (IADLs) should be done on all nonacute elderly patients. USMLE may not employ many standardized patients who are actually this old but may try to make some older adults look elderly. If the Doorway Information gives the patient's age as 90, approach the case as if the patient is 90 whether they look it or not.

ADLs	IADLs
Eating	Cooking
Bathing	Cleaning
Dressing	Doing laundry
Toileting	Shopping
Transferring (e.g., moving from bed to wheelchair)	Using the telephone
	Accessing means of transportation
	Taking medications
	Managing money

Never assume that the problem is just "old age." Alzheimer's disease, depression, stroke, and thyroid disease, as well as cardiovascular and metabolic problems, may be the cause of this patient's symptoms. In addition, side effects of medications are a huge problem in the elderly, so it will be important to ensure that a detailed medication history is taken (dosages not required).

FROM THE STANDARDIZED PATIENT

History

HPI: David Miller Sr. has not been in for a visit in about a year. He says he has run out of his medication, and his son insisted he come in to see the doctor. The patient moved in with his son, David Miller Jr., last year after having lived alone for 20 years. David Sr. had always been fiercely independent, but 2 years ago David Jr. began to worry about his father's increasing forgetfulness. When asked what makes his son worry, the patient admits that on one occasion he left the stove on and twice he'd gotten lost taking a walk around the neighborhood he had known for 20 years. He also says he bounced a few checks and his son "made a federal case of it."

A year ago David Sr. had a stroke, but the weakness in the left side of his body resolved completely. After that, he agreed to move in with his son. The patient admits he has "slowed down" in recent months. He has lost his interest in reading but attributes that to the internet ruining the book industry: "There are no more good books to read." He is starting to need some help with bathing. He dresses and eats independently but has a poor appetite much of the time. When asked about his mood, he admits to crying sometimes, wondering whether he's lived too long, since so many of his friends and family from his generation are gone. This makes him sentimental and inclined to talk about his platoon when he was in Korea in 1950.

Allergies: PCN

Medications: Lisinopril, ASA

PMH: Hospitalized—for stroke 1 year ago. Illness—HTN for 10 years controlled with lisinopril; osteoarthritis. No trauma. Surgery—appendicitis at age 23, transurethral resection of the prostate (TURP) at age 68. No recent surgery.

Review of Symptoms: No trouble urinating. Sleeps about 4 hours during the day. Has trouble sleeping at night.

Diet: States nothing tastes good; complains of constipation.

Social Hx: Has not smoked in last 30 years. Drinks 1 oz whiskey every evening to sleep. Worked as a journalist for 30 years. In retirement, taught underprivileged children to read.

Mental Status Exam

Current month: Incorrect; patient names a month two months prior.

Current year: Patient stumbles, then corrects himself. ("Nineteen . . . I mean, 2017.")

Day: Incorrect; patient is one day off.

Date: Incorrect

Season: Correct

President: Correct

Location: Incorrect. Patient answers, "In your office." If asked where is the office, patient says, "Right here in the city." If still asked which city, the patient hesitates and changes the subject.

State: Correct

Three words: Remembers only two out of three.

Spell "world" backwards: Incorrect. Spells it forwards correctly and backwards incorrectly.

Repeat "no ifs, ands, or buts": Correct.

Read instruction and then do what it says ("Close your eyes"): Patient closes eyes.

Listen to a sentence and write it down ("You are a nice doctor"): Patient does correctly.

Three-stage command: The patient does the first two commands but forgets what the third one was.

Name these items: Correct; patient can name all three.

THE CLOSING

As with all cases, it is important to explain your clinical impression to your patient and discuss the next steps in working up the condition. If you need to gather more information from another source like an adult child, it's important to get the patient's permission to do so.

> **Doctor:** "Mr. Miller, let me summarize what you've told me and make sure I understand. It seems like you've had some trouble with your memory for over a year now. In addition, you've been without your blood pressure medication for a while. More recently, you are struggling with a decline in your mood."
>
> **Mr. Miller:** "Well, I'm 90. Doesn't that happen to everyone at my age?"
>
> **Doctor:** "While these are common problem for people your age, we should do some tests to make sure that there isn't something else that we could treat. I also would like to speak to your son and help you both to figure out how to get whatever help you might need at home. Is that okay with you?"

SAMPLE PATIENT NOTE

History: Describe the history you just obtained from this patient. Include only information (pertinent positives and negatives) relevant to this patient's problem(s).

CC: *Patient is unable to care for himself.*

HPI: *David Miller Sr., 90 years old, has increasing forgetfulness, decreasing ability to self-care, and increasing difficulty with IADs and some ADLs. Started 2–3 years ago with forgetfulness. Unable to do his own banking. For last year has lived with his son but is increasingly "slowed down." Episodes of crying. Has lost interest in reading, despite former career as journalist. In past months has increasing difficulty in preparing meals, eating, and hygiene. Denies suicidal ideation but admits sleep disturbance and poor appetite. Reversal of day/night sleep cycle. Out of HTN meds for several months.*

Medications: Lisinopril, ASA

ROS: *No change in urination. + constipation.*

PMH: *Hospitalizations for stroke 1 year ago, HTN. No trauma. Previous appendectomy at age 23. TURP at age 68.*

SH: *Lives with son, denies tobacco for past 30 years. Pt has 1 oz whiskey every evening.*

SAMPLE PATIENT NOTE

Physical Examination: Describe any positive and negative findings relevant to this patient's problem(s). Be careful to include *only* those parts of examination you performed in *this* encounter.

BP: *165/85 mm Hg*

Mental
status
exam: *Markedly abnormal with only partial orientation to place, disorientation to date.*

Remembers only 2/3 items at 5 minutes.

Spells "world" forward correctly, unable to spell it backwards.

Naming and writing intact and without dysarthria.

Follows only 2 commands when given 3 commands.

SAMPLE PATIENT NOTE

Data Interpretation: *Based on what you have learned from the history and physical examination,* list up to 3 diagnoses that might explain this patient's complaint(s). List your diagnoses from most to least likely. For some cases, fewer than 3 diagnoses will be appropriate. Then, enter the positive or negative findings from the history and the physical examination (if present) that support each diagnosis. Lastly, list initial *diagnostic* studies (if any) you would order for this patient (e.g., restricted physical exam maneuvers, laboratory tests, imaging, ECG, etc.).

Diagnosis #1: Dementia from Alzheimer's

Differential diagnosis and diagnostic reasoning

History Finding(s)

Progressive inability to self-care

Deficits in IADs, some ADLs

Decline in mental abilities over 2–3 years: leaving stove on, getting lost in own neighborhood

Physical Exam Finding(s)

MSE deficits in memory, attention, and orientation

Diagnosis #2: Multi-infarct dementia

Differential diagnosis and diagnostic reasoning

History Finding(s)

History of stroke in past

Physical Exam Finding(s)

MSE deficits as noted

Diagnosis #3: Pseudodementia from depression

Differential diagnosis and diagnostic reasoning

History Finding(s)

Episodes of crying

Loss of interest, poor appetite

Feels slowed down

Alteration in sleep habits

Physical Exam Finding(s)

Decreased attention on MSE

Diagnostic Study/Studies

CBC, lytes, BUN, Cr, glucose

MRI of brain

TSH, VDRL

B12, folate level

CASE DISCUSSION

Notes about the History-Taking

This is a case where involving the family will be key. Getting potentially more reliable information from close family (son) and involving them in management will be essential. With all cases of memory loss, reduced functioning, or depressed mood in the elderly, expect to undertake mental status exam and functional assessment (ADLs and IADs).

Comments about the Patient Note

The workup for dementia that's listed here is fairly standard, and you can use it for any older person with confusion or mental status changes.

This is a very difficult case with a broad differential. Try to write down the diagnoses most likely based on the history and physical.

Case 14: **Abdominal Pain and Fatigue**

DOORWAY INFORMATION

Opening Scenario

Kim Turner is a 29 y/o female with 2 months of abdominal pain, fatigue, and just not feeling well. This is her third visit in 2 months.

Vital Signs

- Temp: 37.0°C (98.6°F)
- BP: 120/80 mm Hg
- HR: 80/min
- RR: 16/min

Examinee Tasks

1. Obtain a focused history.
2. Perform a relevant physical examination. Do not perform rectal, pelvic, genitourinary, inguinal hernia, female breast, or corneal reflex examinations.
3. Discuss your initial diagnostic impression and your workup plan with the patient.
4. After leaving the room, complete your patient note on the given form.

BEFORE ENTERING THE ROOM

Clinical Reasoning: There could be several reasons why a patient makes multiple return visits. This patient presents with an acute problem each visit. The multiple visits could be just following up at the doctor's request after test results are back or treatment is reevaluated. The underlying condition may be something unusual that has so far eluded diagnosis. Or there may be a social problem that has yet to be elucidated. The history will require you to ask some direct and possibly sensitive questions.

Fatigue is a common symptom and there are many conditions to consider. Any chronic illness can make a patient fatigued. Doing a thyroid exam, ordering a TSH and using hypothyroidism as a diagnosis will always be correct in this situation. Also consider anemia, diabetes, and depression as additional common problems.

You may not yet know the cause of this patient's abdominal pain but one of the first things you should recognize before entering the room is that her vital signs are stable. With 2 months of pain and currently normal vital signs, it is not likely that this is going to be an acute abdomen or a surgical problem. You should be deducing a differential diagnosis that helps to explain all (or almost all) of the patient's symptoms.

FROM THE STANDARDIZED PATIENT

History

HPI: Ms. Turner states that she has had abdominal pain off and on for the past 6 months. It started slowly, and can last anywhere from minutes to days. It can occur in any or multiple quadrants of her abdomen. It feels crampy. It is 10/10 when it happens. Other times, the pain is milder. It never radiates to the back or groin. She sometimes takes a lorazepam tablet (benzodiazepine), which seems to help. She was given the lorazepam for sleep a couple of years ago in the hospital.

The pain is significantly aggravated when she is not getting along with her son's father, especially after they argue. No fever, chills, anorexia, vomiting, diarrhea, jaundice, or dysuria. Prior to the last 6 months, she has not had any problems with abdominal pain.

Ms. Turner takes lorazepam now and then when she feels really fatigued and not well and on nights when she can't fall asleep. In general, she is not sleeping well and wakes up frequently. Her weight and diet have not changed.

She was hospitalized in the past for a blowout fracture of the orbit a couple of years ago when she tripped off a curb. Last year she was hospitalized for "some bleeding inside." She carries the hospital discharge papers with her. She hands you a paper that says "Idiopathic retroperitoneal hemorrhage." If you ask about trauma, she will tell you "No" at this point. There is no family history of hemophilia or bleeding disorder.

Her last menstrual period was 2 weeks ago and was normal. She is G2P2. Her youngest child is 7 years old. She is sexually active with her son's father when he stays with them. She does use the Pill. She has never had a sexually transmitted disease. Her son's father lives about half the year with them and spends a lot of time somewhere else. She is chronically stressed about the relationship.

Social Hx: She smokes 1 pack per day. Denies alcohol or recreational drugs.

PMH: No surgery other than to reconstruct her face.

Meds: Lorazepam, ibuprofen as needed.

Physical Exam

Patient appears to be in no acute distress, although she is not smiling. Her head is normocephalic. She does still have some chronic pain in the cheek where her facial bones were broken, but says that it's a lot better and healing well. Her pharynx is normal. Her neck is supple.

Chest: There are ecchymoses on her anterior chest wall. Her respiratory excursion is normal. There is tenderness to the left posterior ribs with additional ecchymosis. Percussion, tactile fremitus, and auscultation of the lungs are normal. If asked, she says it does hurt when she takes a deep breath. Her heart tones are normal.

Abdomen: Free of any rash or ecchymosis. Bowel sounds are normal. Her abdomen is a little tender all along the left side. No rebound. There is no CVA tenderness. Her extremities appear normal. She is alert. Her gait is normal. Motor strength is equal in all four extremities. She denies feeling sad, helpless, or hopeless.

THE CLOSING

Doctor: "Ms. Turner, you told me you have this abdominal pain. On your exam I found you are tender in the belly and have large bruises on your chest. I am concerned that when you were injured you may have hurt your chest or belly. Ms. Turner, many women are victims of domestic violence. If anyone is hurting you, we can help get to a place that is safe. I know it's difficult to talk about. No one has the right to hurt you."

Ms. Turner: "He is really a good man. But sometimes he loses his temper."

Doctor: "I'd like you to see our counselor to help. Also I want to be sure you have a safe place to go when you feel you are in danger."

SAMPLE PATIENT NOTE

History: Describe the history you just obtained from this patient. Include only information (pertinent positives and negatives) relevant to this patient's problem(s).

CC: Fatigue, weakness, abdominal pain for 2 months

HPI: 29 y/o female states has intermittent abdominal pain for 2 months. It can last hours to days and is migratory to all 4 Q. Described as crampy, mild to severe in nature. Better when she takes Ativan, worse with arguing with her son's father. No diarrhea, vomiting, anorexia, fever, dysuria, or jaundice.

               Lives with son. Son's father in household about ½ time. Stressed over relationship. Admits to domestic violence from son's father. Fractured orbit 2 years ago and hx of "idiopathic retroperitoneal hemorrhage" last year.

               Denies SOB or chest pain. She denies feeling sad, hopeless, or guilty. Has not been sleeping well, no recent change in weight.

               Meds: Oral contraceptives, lorazepam

PMH: No prior episodes

Family Hx: No hx of bleeding disorder

SX: Active, one partner. No hx of STD. LMP 2 wks ago NL. G2P2.

SH: + Smokes. − Drugs/alcohol.

SAMPLE PATIENT NOTE

Physical Examination: Describe any positive and negative findings relevant to this patient's problem(s). Be careful to include *only* those parts of examination you performed in *this* encounter.

VS: 37.0 120/80 80 16

GA: NAD. Pt not smiling.

HEENT: PEERL, pharynx clear. Some tenderness remains on face from old fracture. Thyroid: Not enlarged, without tenderness.

Chest: Bruise along L thoracic posterior ribs. Mildly tender, NL respiratory excursion. No flail chest. Normal, fremitus, percussion, and auscultation. Also bruise on anterior chest wall.

Abd: No ecchymosis. BS+, mild LUQ, LLQ tenderness. No mass or rebound. No CVA pain.

Extremities: Appear NL

SAMPLE PATIENT NOTE

Data Interpretation: Based on what you have learned from the history and physical examination, list up to 3 diagnoses that might explain this patient's complaint(s). List your diagnoses from most to least likely. For some cases, fewer than 3 diagnoses will be appropriate. Then, enter the positive or negative findings from the history and the physical examination (if present) that support each diagnosis. Lastly, list initial diagnostic studies (if any) you would order for this patient (e.g., restricted physical exam maneuvers, laboratory tests, imaging, ECG, etc.).

Diagnosis #1: Domestic violence

Differential diagnosis and diagnostic reasoning

History Finding(s)	**Physical Exam Finding(s)**
Patient admits to being abused	Multiple unexplained bruises

Diagnosis #2: Hemopneumothorax

Differential diagnosis and diagnostic reasoning

History Finding(s)	**Physical Exam Finding(s)**
Admits to being abused and gives hx of retroperitoneal hemorrhage	Bruised and tender L post-thoracic ribs

Diagnosis #3: Traumatic injury of spleen

Differential diagnosis and diagnostic reasoning

History Finding(s)	**Physical Exam Finding(s)**
Blunt trauma	Tender in LUQ

Diagnostic Study/Studies

Pelvic and rectal exam

CBC, INR

CXR, U/A

CT Abd

CASE DISCUSSION

Notes about the History-Taking

The patient will not tell you about domestic violence unless you express empathy and understanding and talk about confidentiality and safety.

1. Empathy: If the SP feels that you are not caring, the SP will not admit to the domestic violence.
2. Statement of confidentiality: Somewhere in the interview (preferably sooner rather than later), inform the patient that the interview is confidential. Some states have mandatory reporting laws, but since Step 2 CS is a national exam, it is unlikely to require you to address that.
3. Safety statement: You must speak to the patient's unmentioned concern about her safety. You must tell the patient that you can put her in touch with resources that can help keep her safe.

Notes about the Physical Exam

Once you find the bruise on the anterior chest, you should realize it is necessary to check the entire body for additional simulated physical findings. Also, a bruise over the chest would indicate that you should do as complete a chest exam as time will allow.

It is necessary to ask additional history during the physical exam when you find the rather dramatic bruising. Ask about chest pain and shortness of breath. You will also want to ask how the fresh bruises got there.

Be sure to consider physical injuries on a domestic violence case.

Patients with normal vital signs can still have an injury of the spleen.

Comments about the Patient Note

If the patient will not admit to the diagnosis of domestic violence, you can still use it as a differential diagnosis. Write "Suspect domestic violence."

Certainly, the focus in a domestic violence case is not only to arrange for counseling but also to diagnose and work up any injuries.

Case 15: **Child with Vomiting and Diarrhea**

DOORWAY INFORMATION

Opening Scenario

Ashley Martin is an 18-month-old female child whose mother wishes to talk to you about the child's vomiting and diarrhea.

Vital Signs

There are no vital signs taken in this case.

Examinee Tasks

1. Obtain a focused history.
2. You will not be required to perform a physical examination in this case.
3. Discuss your initial diagnostic impression and your workup plan with the patient.
4. After leaving the room, complete your patient note on the given form.

BEFORE ENTERING THE ROOM

Clinical Reasoning: There will be no child SPs present on test day. Pediatric cases will be represented via a surrogate (a parent or caretaker who will speak with you in person or by phone). Since you will not be required to complete a physical exam during the encounter, you may spend the extra time completing the pediatric history.

Diarrhea may have several different causes: bacterial infection, parasitic infections, medications, or viral diarrhea.

This case is intended to test your ability to obtain a history that helps elucidate the cause of the vomiting and diarrhea. In addition, you will need to ask questions that may help you determine the severity of the child's condition, and make a triage decision as to whether the child needs to be seen, and with what urgency, and provide guidance to the parent/caregiver.

FROM THE MOTHER

History

HPI: Mrs. Martin calls you to tell you that her 18-month-old child is sick. It started about 48 hours ago with vomiting and fussiness. Ashley has thrown up a total of 3 times a day for the past 2 days. The vomiting began with food. Now just water and mucus is coming up, as the baby will not eat or drink much. For the past day, Ashley has had 4 episodes of diarrhea. The diarrhea is brown and watery. She seems to be hot, but Mrs. Martin does not have a thermometer and has not taken her temperature. At times, especially when she is having a bowel movement, the baby appears to be in pain. Ashley won't smile or play, seems to be more tired than usual, and has not had a wet diaper from urine in 8 hours. Mrs. Martin isn't sure if any diapers contained both urine and stool due to the large amount of diarrhea. (She needed a quick bath after each episode of diarrhea, and her bottom is looking red already.) When the child cries, there are tears.

This all began 3 days after returning from a play-date with a group of other toddlers. Acetaminophen seems to make Ashley feel a little better, but the vomiting and diarrhea have not stopped. Drinking cow's milk seems to make the diarrhea worse, when the child is less active and playful. She prefers to sit quietly and watch TV. Constantly, she wants to be held and rocked gently. There is no rash or yellowing of the skin. No cough or runny nose, no shortness of breath. Still, Mrs. Martin is worried that Ashley does not look so good.

Ashley has never had this before. She finished a course of amoxicillin for otitis media just as the fever and vomiting began. She has a greatly decreased appetite and has not been sleeping well. There is no travel history. No one else in the family has a similar illness.

Ped Hx: Mrs. Martin received prenatal care while pregnant with Ashley and did not smoke or use drugs or alcohol. She carried Ashley to full term but had a C-section after a 28-hour labor. Ashley had no problems in the first days and weeks of life. She was breastfed for the first 8 months. Now she eats regular table food and cow's milk. Growth and development are normal. She started walking at 1 year and was just starting to urinate in the potty during the daytime when she got sick. She gets regular checkups. Her immunizations are complete.

Meds: She has no known allergies to medication or food. Aside from pediatric vitamins, she takes no meds.

PMH: She has had no hospitalizations, other than at birth for 24 hours. No surgery, major illnesses, or trauma.

Social Hx: Ashley lives with her mother, father, and a golden retriever dog.

Physical Exam

There is no physical exam in this case.

THE CLOSING

Doctor: "Mrs. Martin, thank you for calling me today about Ashley. Let me make sure I understand. On the last day of the amoxicillin that she was taking for an ear infection, she started with fever and vomiting. That was 2 days ago. Then yesterday she started with diarrhea. There are a few possibilities. She could have a new infection, probably a virus, making her sick, or her symptoms may also be from the antibiotics. Either way, my concern is that she could be getting dehydrated. If she can't keep fluids down, she may need to receive fluids through an intravenous line. I'd like you to stop milk for now and instead give her fluids such as Pedialyte, which will help. I will also need to see her as soon as possible for an exam. Can you bring her in to see me now?"

The key here is that you're always available and you want to see the patient. If it sounds like a medical emergency, have her call 9-1-1 and tell her you will meet her at the hospital. In pediatrics, you generally want to see the child for any illness *today*.

CHALLENGING QUESTIONS

Mrs. Martin: "Oh, I have no transportation and can't come today."

Doctor: "Hmmm. It sounds like I need to see Ashley today. I need to examine her to make sure nothing more serious is going on. Can you take a taxi or ask someone to drive you? If you cannot come in right away, please call the ambulance and have them bring you into the emergency room. I will meet you there."

SAMPLE PATIENT NOTE

History: Describe the history you just obtained from this patient. Include only information (pertinent positives and negatives) relevant to this patient's problem(s).

CC: 18-month-old with vomiting and diarrhea

HPI: 2 days of vomiting and being fussy and febrile. Vomited 6 times total, first just food, now clear. No blood. 1 day of diarrhea, 4 episodes, brown and watery. Seems to have cramps with BM. Fever better with acetaminophen. Diarrhea worse when drinks milk. No cough, coryza, dysuria, or rash. Decreased play, more lethargic than usual. No difficulty with arousal. No sick contacts or travel history. No prior episodes of vomiting and diarrhea. Diarrhea started after a course of antibiotics for otitis media. Child has decreased appetite and not sleeping well. Breast-fed until 8 mo, now on regular food and cow's milk. Mom states growth and development are normal.

Uncomplicated perinatal course.

Allergies: NKMA

Meds: Pediatric vitamins. Tylenol for fever. Recent course of amoxicillin for otitis media.

PMH: No hospitalization, surgery, trauma, or major illness.

SH: Ashley lives with parents and dog.

SAMPLE PATIENT NOTE

Physical Examination: Describe any positive and negative findings relevant to this patient's problem(s). Be careful to include *only* those parts of examination you performed in *this* encounter.

There is no physical exam in this case.

SAMPLE PATIENT NOTE

Data Interpretation: *Based on what you have learned from the history and physical examination,* list up to 3 diagnoses that might explain this patient's complaint(s). List your diagnoses from most to least likely. For some cases, fewer than 3 diagnoses will be appropriate. Then, enter the positive or negative findings from the history and the physical examination (if present) that support each diagnosis. Lastly, list initial *diagnostic* studies (if any) you would order for this patient (e.g., restricted physical exam maneuvers, laboratory tests, imaging, ECG, etc.).

Diagnosis #1: Dehydration

Differential diagnosis and diagnostic reasoning

History Finding(s)   Physical Exam Finding(s)

Vomiting and diarrhea, poor po intake

Decreased play, seems lethargic

Diagnosis #2: Gastroenteritis

Differential diagnosis and diagnostic reasoning

History Finding(s)   Physical Exam Finding(s)

Vomiting and diarrhea

Pt holding abdomen, appears to be in
pain per mother's report

Diagnosis #3: Diarrhea from amoxicillin

Differential diagnosis and diagnostic reasoning

History Finding(s)   Physical Exam Finding(s)

Diarrhea began right after course of
amoxicillin

Diagnostic Study/Studies

Physical exam

U/A

Lytes, glucose, BUN

Stool for C-diff

CASE DISCUSSION

Notes about the History-Taking

Emphasis here is given on getting the number of times—and the color—of the vomiting and diarrhea. Since you cannot "see" your patient, it's helpful to get a description of the child's activity level. Is the baby floppy or listless? Is she interactive with her environment? Clues to dehydration are lack of wet diapers; more severe dehydration can cause a lack of tears when child is crying. A complete pediatric history will be expected on children younger than 2 years of age.

Notes about the Physical Exam

There was no physical exam in this case.

Case 16: **Fatigue**

DOORWAY INFORMATION

Opening Scenario

John Brown is a 55 y/o male who comes to the office wanting a physical exam, complaining of fatigue.

Vital Signs

- Temp: 37.0°C (98.6°F)
- BP: 130/70 mm Hg, right upper limb sitting
- HR: 90/min, regular
- RR: 20/min

Examinee Tasks

1. Obtain a focused history.
2. Perform a relevant physical examination. Do not perform rectal, pelvic, genitourinary, inguinal hernia, female breast, or corneal reflex examinations.
3. Discuss your initial diagnostic impression and your workup plan with the patient.
4. After leaving the room, complete the standard patient form that is waiting for you at your desk.

BEFORE ENTERING THE ROOM

Clinical Reasoning: When the chief complaint is vague and not really related to a specific organ system, the differential will likely include multiple systems. The first question to ask about fatigue is to assess sleep, as disrupted sleep is the most common cause. In addition, you need to distinguish sleepiness from lack of exercise tolerance. Other diagnoses can present with fatigue include diabetes, thyroid disease (hypo or hyper), anemia, depression, heart failure, and malignancy.

FROM THE STANDARDIZED PATIENT

History

HPI: Mr. Brown says he has been fatigued for the past 2 months. He's given up exercise and has trouble getting out of bed in the morning. He has little energy for anything besides going to work. No unusual stress, he says. He denies having any shortness of breath, chest pain, or blood in the stool. No chronic cough, no sores that won't heal, and no fevers, hoarseness, or trouble swallowing. He has no trouble falling asleep and sleeps for a total of 8 hours a night but wakes up a few times to urinate—he has been urinating a lot at night as well as during the daytime. He drinks a lot of bottled water because he is frequently thirsty. No burning with urination, no blood in the urine, and no disturbance in flow of urine or hesitancy. He is taking saw palmetto to help with a problem of frequent urination.

Mr. Brown reports feeling cold often and when others aren't. He has intermittent blurry vision but denies any numbness or weakness. He thinks he is eating more, but his weight has not changed in the past 2 months. His diet consists of high-carbohydrate, high-fat meals, and he admits to eating a lot of fast food. He has gained about 50 lb. in the last 5 years. He denies drinking coffee and tea but does drink sodas.

He has not been sexually active recently. Has had problems maintaining an erection.

Mr. Brown had his gallbladder removed 5 years ago. That was the last time he had his blood pressure or any blood tests taken. He denies diabetes, hypertension, or heart disease.

FH: Dad and older brother died at age 58 of heart attack. Brother has diabetes.

Social Hx: Lives with his wife. No recreational drug use. Has smoked 1 pack per day for the past 20 years. EtOH: has one or two drinks three times a week. Works as an air traffic controller.

Physical Exam

Mr. Brown states his weight is 100 kg. He is 5 feet, 6 inches tall. He is in no distress. His vision is 20/30 in both eyes. His pupils are normal, and reactive to light. The fundoscopic exam reveals a normal red reflex. His pharynx is normal. His neck exam reveals no carotid bruits or thyromegaly. He has no jugular venous distention. His nail beds appear pink. His lungs are clear to auscultation on both sides. His heart sounds are normal. There are no rubs or murmurs heard. You cannot feel the point of maximum impulse, perhaps due to his obesity. His belly is soft, obese, nontender, and without masses. An old scar from the gall bladder surgery is located in the right subcostal abdomen. He has some edema of both lower extremities. Distal pulses are equal and strong in the hands and feet. Mr. Brown is alert. He is able to walk normally. His strength is equal and strong in all 4 extremities. There is no redness or tenderness or open sores on the feet. He has decreased sensation to light touch in both feet below the ankles.

THE CLOSING

As with all cases, it is important to explain your clinical impression to your patient and discuss the next steps in working up his condition.

> **Doctor:** "All right, Mr. Brown. Let me just summarize what you have described to me. You have been very fatigued for the last two months and had weight gain over the last few years, a thirsty feeling, and the need to urinate frequently. You have a family history of diabetes.
>
> "I'd like to see if you have high blood sugar and run some basic tests for your heart, thyroid, and blood counts. Also, for your ongoing health, I would recommend that you stop smoking. Quitting cigarettes is the single most important thing you can do for your health, as it prevents a large number of health conditions. I know that we've discussed a lot today, but I want to make sure that you understand all of these things. Do you have questions for me?"

SAMPLE PATIENT NOTE

History: Describe the history you just obtained from this patient. Include only information (pertinent positives and negatives) relevant to this patient's problem(s).

CC: 55 y/o male presenting with 2 months of fatigue

HPI: Mr. Brown c/o fatigue, has noticed increased frequency of urination. Also frequently thirsty and has 50-lb weight gain in 5 years. No dysuria or hematuria. No SOB, chest pain, cough, hoarseness, change in bowel habits, or blood in stool. Some sensory changes, intermittent blurry vision. Sleeping 8 hours a night but gets up secondary to nocturia. His weight has stabilized despite eating more. Stopped exercising since he's too tired. Has cold intolerance, erectile dysfunction. Family history of diabetes.

Allergies: None

Meds: None

PMH: Hospitalized for cholecystectomy 5 yrs ago. No hx DM, no reported hx HTN. Never had sugar checked.

ROS: Diet—fast food, high fat.

SH: Lives with wife. Smokes 1 ppd, EtOH 1–2 drinks 3x/wk. No drug use. States no unusual stresses.

SAMPLE PATIENT NOTE

Physical Examination: Describe any positive and negative findings relevant to this patient's problem(s). Be careful to include *only* those parts of examination you performed in *this* encounter.

VS: 90 20 98.6 BP = 130/70. Ht 5 ft 6 in, wt 220 lb.

GA: No distress

HEENT: PERRL, V/A 20/30 OU. Fundi: NL red reflex. No thyromegaly, − JVD.

Chest: Lungs clear to A B/L

CV: S2: WNL, PMI not palpable.

Abd: Soft, obese, nontender. No masses. Old R subcostal scar.

Neuro: Gait NL, motor 5/5 all 4 ext, decreased light touch below ankle B/L.

SAMPLE PATIENT NOTE

Data Interpretation: *Based on what you have learned from the history and physical examination,* list up to 3 diagnoses that might explain this patient's complaint(s). List your diagnoses from most to least likely. For some cases, fewer than 3 diagnoses will be appropriate. Then, enter the positive or negative findings from the history and the physical examination (if present) that support each diagnosis. Lastly, list initial *diagnostic* studies (if any) you would order for this patient (e.g., restricted physical exam maneuvers, laboratory tests, imaging, ECG, etc.).

Diagnosis #1: Diabetes

Differential diagnosis and diagnostic reasoning

History Finding(s)	Physical Exam Finding(s)
Polyuria, polydipsia, fatigue, nocturia	Decreased sensation feet
Weight not increasing though eating more	Obese
Blurry vision, erectile dysfunction	
Family history of DM	

Diagnosis #2: Hypothyroidism

Differential diagnosis and diagnostic reasoning

History Finding(s)	Physical Exam Finding(s)
50-lb weight gain in 5 years	
Fatigue	
Cold intolerance	

Diagnosis #3: Anemia

Differential diagnosis and diagnostic reasoning

History Finding(s)	Physical Exam Finding(s)
Fatigue	Decreased sensation below knees B/L to light touch
Cold intolerance	
Decreased exercise tolerance	

Diagnostic Study/Studies

Rectal and prostate exam

CBC, U/A, TSH

Electrolytes, BUN, Cr

HgA1c

Fasting glucose

CASE DISCUSSION

Comments about the Note

Even though you may not find out about Mr. Brown's many symptoms until the ROS questions, it is fine to include this information in the HPI of the Patient Note. This will demonstrate that you are able to organize information from the patient history into a logical patient note, and shows the graders the important features that support your primary diagnosis, which, in this case, is diabetes.

Case 17: **Obesity**

DOORWAY INFORMATION

Opening Scenario

Susan Adams is an 18 y/o female who has come to the clinic concerned about her weight gain.

Vital Signs

- Temp: 37.0°C (98.6°F)
- BP: 130/80 mm Hg, right upper limb sitting
- HR: 85/min, regular
- RR: 14/min
- Weight 220 lb., BMI 39

Examinee Tasks

1. Obtain a focused history.
2. Since this is largely a counseling case, you will not be required to perform a physical examination.
3. Discuss your initial diagnostic impression and your workup plan with the patient.
4. After leaving the room, complete your patient note on the given form.

BEFORE ENTERING THE ROOM

Clinical Reasoning: The opening scenario gives you information (patient's BMI) that can begin your thinking about the case, but you must keep an open mind as to what this entire case is about. You will need to order a physical exam on the patient note and you will need to take an adolescent history. As with any adolescent patient case, remember to give a message of confidentiality early in the encounter.

Keep in mind that obesity is associated with depression and eating disorders, so you should ask about symptoms of depression. Obesity is often a cause for shame in patients so you must be very careful to be sensitive about attributing any blame and be empathic about how hard the patient has struggled. Avoid using the terms *obese* and *obesity* with patients.

There is an obesity epidemic in the United States. It is mainly attributed to large portions of high-calorie foods (high-fat and high-sugar meals) and a sedentary lifestyle. Secondary causes of obesity may also be considered, such as hypothyroidism, insulinoma, Cushing syndrome, and polycystic ovarian disease; however, these account for a small fraction of the total number of cases.

FROM THE PATIENT

History

HPI: When she tells you about her weight problem, Susan says she feels defeated by the number of diets she has attempted, and she appears to have given up on her weight loss. Susan is 5 feet 2 inches and 220 lb. She would like you to recommend a diet. Since the age of 8 months, Susan has always been above the 95th percentile for weight on the growth charts. By second grade she was the heaviest child in her class, and she has remained so throughout her life. She has tried various popular commercial diets, but at best they helped her to maintain the same weight for a few months. When she stopped a certain diet, her weight would typically increase.

Susan carries most of her weight around her belly. She has a very negative body image, and it is affecting her self-esteem. She has not had many friends in high school and has not been asked to prom. Susan says she is sad and hopeless about her condition. She has never thought of harming herself, but she frequently stands in front of the refrigerator and eats for hours into the night. Susan recognizes that she often eats when bored, dissatisfied, or depressed. She has less energy than usual lately. She never tries to make herself vomit.

Susan has been sleeping more than usual lately. Her diet consists mostly of high-fat and processed foods. She eats many crackers, but few fruits and vegetables.

Susan had menarche at age 15 and gets her period only once every few months. That is another thing that she is concerned about. Susan is not sexually active. Susan is also very self-conscious about the fact that she has some facial hair and bad acne.

Susan lives at home with her mother and father. She is a senior in high school with average grades. She works on the yearbook as her only extracurricular activity. She does not drink alcohol, use drugs, or smoke cigarettes.

PHM: Susan has never been hospitalized. No surgery or trauma. Never diagnosed with diabetes. She takes no medications.

Family Hx: Susan says that everyone in her family is a little overweight.

Physical Exam

There is no physical exam in this case.

THE CLOSING

Doctor: "Thank you for coming to talk to me today, Susan. It sounds like you have been struggling with your weight your entire life. Now it is affecting your self-esteem, and you are also worried about having very irregular menstrual periods. I'd like to do a physical exam and order some blood tests to make sure that you don't have any medical problems that are causing or a result of your weight gain. There are many conditions that can cause one to be overweight."

CHALLENGING QUESTIONS

Susan: "I've read about some prescription pills for weight loss. Can't you just give me a prescription?"

Doctor: "Those pills only work in the short term, and they come with many risks and side effects. Once I've done a physical examination and reviewed your blood work, we can talk about the best options for you."

SAMPLE PATIENT NOTE

History: Describe the history you just obtained from this patient. Include only information (pertinent positives and negatives) relevant to this patient's problem(s).

CC: 18 y/o female with weight gain/obesity

HPI: Pt has been above 95% for weight her entire life. Now 5'2", 220 lb., BMI 39. Has tried multiple commercial diets without success. Pt has poor body image. Frequently eats large amounts of food late into the night; triggers include boredom and feelings of hopelessness. Her diet consists of few fruits and vegetables and mostly high-fat processed foods and crackers. Has decreased energy. No hx of self-harm ideation. Sleeping more than usual lately. Is an average student, a senior in high school. No recent change in grades. Does not have many friends. Pt embarrassed about acne and facial hair. Menarche age 15, periods very irregular. Not sexually active. Many overweight family members. Lives with mother and father. Does not smoke or use alcohol or drugs.

Meds: None

PMH: No hospitalizations, trauma, or surgery. No hx of DM, HTN.

SAMPLE PATIENT NOTE

Physical Examination: Describe any positive and negative findings relevant to this patient's problem(s). Be careful to include *only* those parts of examination you performed in *this* encounter.

There is no physical exam in this case.

SAMPLE PATIENT NOTE

Data Interpretation: *Based on what you have learned from the history and physical examination,* list up to 3 diagnoses that might explain this patient's complaint(s). List your diagnoses from most to least likely. For some cases, fewer than 3 diagnoses will be appropriate. Then, enter the positive or negative findings from the history and the physical examination (if present) that support each diagnosis. Lastly, list initial *diagnostic* studies (if any) you would order for this patient (e.g., restricted physical exam maneuvers, laboratory tests, imaging, ECG, etc.).

Diagnosis #1: Binge eating disorder

Differential diagnosis and diagnostic reasoning

History Finding(s)	Physical Exam Finding(s)
Obesity	
Binge eating at night	

Diagnosis #2: Polycystic ovarian disease

Differential diagnosis and diagnostic reasoning

History Finding(s)	Physical Exam Finding(s)
Amenorrhea	
Obesity/weight gain	
Hirsutism	
Acne	

Diagnosis #3: Hypothyroidism

Differential diagnosis and diagnostic reasoning

History Finding(s)	Physical Exam Finding(s)
Obesity	
Decreased energy level	
Increased sleep requirements	

Diagnostic Study/Studies

Physical exam

TSH, fasting glucose, HgA1c

DHEAS, prolactin level, testosterone level

Ultrasound of the ovaries

CASE DISCUSSION

Notes about the History-Taking

Eating disorders that cause obesity include binge eating disorder and bulimia. They are commonly associated with depression but can occur without depression as well. With all of these disorders, the patient feels unable to control his/her eating. Specific eating disorders may be used as differential diagnoses in the obese patient. Binge eating disorder manifests by eating large amounts of food over a short period of time. Bulimia often causes patients to be overweight despite self-induced vomiting.

You may ask your patients about eating disorders by using the following questions:

- What are your eating patterns?
- Do you ever feel that you cannot stop eating when you want to?
- Do you eat when you feel anxious or feel a loss of control?
- Do you make yourself vomit after eating?

Polycystic ovarian disease typically has a workup to include follicle-stimulating hormone (FSH), luteinizing hormone (LH), and prolactin. The use of abbreviations is acceptable. An ultrasound would look at the ovaries.

Notes about the Physical Exam

There is no physical exam in this case.

Case 18: **Fever in a 70-Year-Old**

BEFORE ENTERING THE ROOM

Clinical Reasoning: With an older patient, make sure you find out about known chronic conditions early in the interview, as you likely need to consider complications of that chronic disease in your differential diagnosis. For example, Parkinson's patients are more prone to aspiration pneumonia than other patients, and complications from parkinsonian medications can also cause fever. In addition, high fever is a more significant finding in an older patient. As we age, the body loses its ability to mount a fever, so the older the patient, the more significant and worrisome a fever of 102°F is.

FROM THE STANDARDIZED PATIENT

History

HPI: Mr. Wilson is a 70-year-old man with a history of Parkinson's disease for 5 years who comes into the office from home with fever for 2 days Tmax to 103°F yesterday. He has a cough productive of yellow sputum. Mild shortness of breath began last week, he believes, after he nearly choked on a piece of apple. Mr. Wilson has not been eating well because of increased drooling and—since the apple episode last week—the fear that he will choke on his food. He has not had any change in his sleep. He complains of difficulty swallowing. Mr. Wilson has also had increasing problems walking over the past 2 weeks and almost fell several times. At that time he also started having visual hallucinations that greatly disturbed his sleep, so he was started on quetiapine. In fact, today he really cannot walk at all and had to be carried into your office due to tremor and weakness. He complains of being very stiff. Acetaminophen controls the fever only for a few hours. He feels like he has been getting sicker every day this week and cannot tell why. He denies chest pain, headache or confusion.

Meds: Amantadine—dose increased one month ago. Levodopa—stopped taking 2 weeks ago because he ran out of medicine. No known drug allergies.

PMH: He was hospitalized for pneumonia 1 year ago, from which he made a full recovery. Mr. Wilson had many concussions in the past from boxing as a young man. No surgical history.

Social Hx: Mr. Wilson lives at home with his wife. He does not smoke or use alcohol.

Physical Exam

When you enter the room, you observe that Mr. Wilson is diaphoretic, lying back. He appears to be very stiff and uncomfortable from tremors. His head is without bruising or tenderness. His pupils are round and reactive to light. Mucous membranes of the mouth and pharynx are very dry. He is alert and oriented to person, place, and time. His neck is rigid with passive movement.

Patient's lungs are clear to auscultation. He has normal respiratory excursion, tactile fremitus, and normal percussion. He is tachycardic. No abnormal heart tones are heard. Abdomen is soft. Bowel sounds are present. There is no suprapubic tenderness or masses. No CVA tenderness.

Mr. Wilson has severe bradykinesia and is too weak to walk. He is rigid in all four extremities with passive movement. His sensation is intact in all four extremities.

THE CLOSING

As with all cases, it is important to explain your clinical impression to your patient and discuss the next steps in working up his condition. You should provide some indication about the length of time he may be unable to walk, as this may affect his transportation and employment options. Be sure to answer any additional concerns he may have.

> **Doctor:** "Mr. Wilson, I have finished my physical exam and would like to discuss what might be causing you to feel sick. You told me you have a high fever with yellow sputum. You ran out of levodopa about 2 weeks ago and now you feel very stiff and can't walk. I think you might have an infection in your chest. Stopping the levodopa might also be part of the problem. I'll need to take a picture of your chest and a sample of blood to look for infection. We can do those tests right now and I should have some answers for you in an hour. Then we will talk about treatment. Do you have any questions?"

CHALLENGING QUESTIONS

Mr. Wilson: "Will I be able to go home?"

Doctor: "What you have may be serious, so I think the best place for you to be is the hospital. But I am going to get you the appropriate treatment and will do everything I can to help."

SAMPLE PATIENT NOTE

History: Describe the history you just obtained from this patient. Include only information (pertinent positives and negatives) relevant to this patient's problem(s).

CC: 70 y/o male. Fever

HPI: Pt with Parkinson's who reports 2 days of fever up to 103°F. Has had a cough productive of yellow sputum after getting a bite of apple "down the wrong pipe" last week. Since then not eating well; some drooling and trouble swallowing. Mildly SOB. No chest pain. Pt also has been getting increasingly stiff, with difficulty walking and almost fell several times. This is because of severe weakness, tremor, and rigidity. He is completely incapacitated and cannot move on his own. This has been for the last week as well. The fever goes down with acetaminophen just for a few hours. Nothing in particular seems to make it worse. Two weeks ago he started having trouble sleeping due to visual hallucinations at night, so was started on quetiapine.

       Meds: Amantadine (dose was recently increased last month). Levodopa (has not taken in 2 weeks because ran out). NKDA.

PMH: Hospitalized for pneumonia last year. Parkinson's for 5 years. Had multiple concussions due to boxing in his youth. No recent trauma. No surgery.

SH: Lives with wife; denies tobacco, EtOH, or drug use

SAMPLE PATIENT NOTE

Physical Examination: Describe any positive and negative findings relevant to this patient's problem(s). Be careful to include *only* those parts of examination you performed in *this* encounter.

VS: 160/114, 110, 24, 102°F

GA: Very rigid, diaphoretic

HEENT: Atraumatic, PERRL. Pharynx very dry. Neck supple.

Chest: Resp excursion NL, fremitus NL, percussion NL. Lungs clear to Auscultation.

CV: Tachycardia, S1 S2 NL

Abd: BS+, nontender all 4 quadrants and suprapubic. No CVA tenderness.

Neuro: Alert and oriented to person, place, and time. Motor hard to test, extremely rigid all 4 extremities to passive movement. + Bradykinesia. Pt too weak to walk. Sensation intact all 4 extremities.

SAMPLE PATIENT NOTE

Data Interpretation: *Based on what you have learned from the history and physical examination,* list up to 3 diagnoses that might explain this patient's complaint(s). List your diagnoses from most to least likely. For some cases, fewer than 3 diagnoses will be appropriate. Then, enter the positive or negative findings from the history and the physical examination (if present) that support each diagnosis. Lastly, list initial *diagnostic* studies (if any) you would order for this patient (e.g., restricted physical exam maneuvers, laboratory tests, imaging, ECG, etc.).

Diagnosis #1: Aspiration pneumonia

Differential diagnosis and diagnostic reasoning

History Finding(s)	Physical Exam Finding(s)
Fever to 103°F	Appears ill
Aspiration of apple, difficulty swallowing	Fever
Yellow sputum	Increased RR
Cough	
Mild SOB	

Diagnosis #2: Neuroleptic malignant syndrome

Differential diagnosis and diagnostic reasoning

History Finding(s)	Physical Exam Finding(s)
Inability to move, rigidity, fever	Fever
2 weeks ago started on quetiapine	Rigidity

Diagnosis #3: Anticholinergic side effects

Differential diagnosis and diagnostic reasoning

History Finding(s)	Physical Exam Finding(s)
Increased dose of amantadine	Increased HR
	Dry pharynx

Diagnostic Study/Studies

CBC, blood culture, sputum culture

CXR

U/A, urine culture

Lytes, BUN, Cr

CPK

CASE DISCUSSION

Notes about the History-Taking

This is a complex history in that the patient has two equally important complaints: pneumonia and the worsening Parkinson's symptoms. Usually the two illnesses portrayed will be related—one being a complication of the other—as it is in this case.

With multiple complaints you may not be able to fully explore each complaint separately. This is sometimes confusing in this patient encounter because you have to make decisions and collect only the most relevant history of each complaint instead of strictly following the mnemonic.

Notes about the Physical Exam

This case demonstrates what to do when an SP is portraying a very ill patient. The history is highly suggestive of pneumonia, yet the SP portraying the case reveals no physical findings of pulmonary consolidation! This can obviously happen in the real clinical setting when the patient is dehydrated. So what you will document is exactly what the real physical findings are, as well as physical findings that are obviously simulated. However, when you get to the diagnosis, put more weight on the history. It is the history that gives you the diagnosis in most cases.

Comments about the Patient Note

This patient has separate issues discussed in the HPI. First is a discussion of his pneumonia-like symptoms with the history of the apple aspiration. Sputum and shortness of breath are used for the associated symptoms of his pneumonia. His other complaint is his worsening Parkinson's symptoms. The onset and course of his slow movement, tremor, and weakness are discussed.

Parkinson's consists of the triad of (1) resting tremor, (2) rigidity, and (3) bradykinesia. Also look for dementia and depression in a Parkinson's case.

The workup of this patient is that of any older person with high fever. Blood, urine, and sputum culture as well as CXR will always be correct. The CPK is to look for muscle destruction, which you would see from increased muscle rigidity associated with neuroleptic malignant syndrome (NMS). NMS can be caused by quetiapine and occurs most commonly in the first 2 weeks. A similar syndrome can be seen in patients who abruptly stop levodopa.

The medication history is very important in this case. Amantadine can also be used to treat Parkinson's, and it has anticholinergic properties.

Case 19: **COPD**

BEFORE ENTERING THE ROOM

Clinical Reasoning: Be sure to make note of the elevated RR given in the doorway vital signs.

Looking at this Doorway Information you should realize that a complete smoking history is needed: when did the patient start to smoke, how many packs/day, number of years he has smoked. You should also find out what the patient has done to stop in the past and how successful he was. It is important to not be judgmental, and to be encouraging of the patient's desire to stop. Tailor your approach to the patient's stage of change. A patient wanting to stop smoking needs help with strategies to quit, not a lecture about the risks of smoking.

In this type of case you will also need to ask if the patient has any symptoms related to complications of smoking, e.g., shortness of breath, weight loss, cough, hemoptysis, and hoarseness, to name a few.

Mr. Black's vital signs show that he is tachypneic but not febrile.

FROM THE STANDARDIZED PATIENT

History

Mr. Black states that his mother died last month from lung cancer and emphysema. He realizes it is time for him to stop smoking.

Patient started smoking when he was 12 years old. By age 18 he was smoking one pack a day. By age 30 he smoked 2 packs/day until now. He has tried to quit several times in the past. He has tried going cold turkey, a nicotine patch, even bupropion a couple of years ago. At the most, he can stop smoking for a week or so before he restarts. He has the most trouble resisting smoking when he is anxious. He has noticed that he has a cough productive of greenish sputum for months at a time most winters. Mr. Black considers this a normal finding for smokers.

It is also affecting his life in that he stopped playing racquetball because he gets too winded and a little wheezy with intense physical exertion. He no longer runs for the commuter train when he is late because it would take the entire ride home to catch his breath. Once the conductor wanted to call an ambulance for him, but Mr. Black refused. He has had no fevers, and he has lost about 10 lb in the last 2 years. He is not on a diet. Occasionally, when he has a hard coughing spell, a tiny streak of blood comes up. He is not hoarse. He has no episodes of chest pain. He did have pneumonia last winter.

Mr. Black takes no medications and has no allergies.

He has never been hospitalized. He has had no trauma or major surgery. No history of DM, HTN, or heart or lung disease. He has never had any exposure to tuberculosis.

Mr. Black lives with his wife of 25 years. He works as a consultant. He states that his job is somewhat stressful, and says that's why he smokes. He does not drink alcohol or use recreational drugs.

Physical Exam

When you walk into the room you will see an SP demonstrating pursed-lip breathing and a prolonged expiratory phase. The SP will probably simulate this physical finding for only the first minute or two of the case. His color is pink. The pharynx is normal. There is no supraclavicular or cervical adenopathy. His chest appears normal. Palpation and respiratory excursion, tactile fremitus, percussion, and auscultation will all be normal. He has no jugular venous distension. His heart tones are regular. There is no cyanosis or peripheral edema. Mr. Black does have clubbing. He is awake and alert.

THE CLOSING

Doctor: "Mr. Black, I have finished your physical exam and would like to talk to you about how you can stop smoking. On your exam I see that you are breathing a little fast at rest. It sounds to me like you are also having some symptoms from smoking: the cough and sputum, the time you had pneumonia, and the short-of-breath feeling that has stopped you from playing racquetball. We need to take a CT scan of your chest, measure your oxygen level, and see how we can improve your exercise capacity. I may have you take a breathing test. I want to see if the smoking has done any damage to the lungs."

CHALLENGING QUESTIONS

Mr. Black: "Do I have emphysema? Am I going to need to walk around with an oxygen tank?"

Doctor: "Once I have the tests back I'll be better able to let you know whether your lung function is decreased. The important thing is to focus on preventing any further damage by quitting smoking now that you are ready to quit."

SAMPLE PATIENT NOTE

History: Describe the history you just obtained from this patient. Include only information (pertinent positives and negatives) relevant to this patient's problem(s).

CC: Dyspnea on exertion, wants to stop smoking

HPI: Pt presents wanting to stop smoking. Has smoked since age 12. ~50 pk-year hx. Has tried nicotine patch and bupropion without success. Feels he smokes due to stress of job.
+ Cough productive of sputum for several months each winter, occasional streak of blood. Had pneumonia last year Rx as outpt.
+ SOB, DOE that prevents exercise
+ 10-lb weight loss,
− Chest pain, hoarseness, fevers

NKMA, no meds

PMH: No hospitalizations, trauma, or surgery.

SH: Lives with wife, works as consultant. No alcohol or recreational drugs.

SAMPLE PATIENT NOTE

Physical Examination: Describe any positive and negative findings relevant to this patient's problem(s). Be careful to include *only* those parts of examination you performed in *this* encounter.

VS: 37.2 130/80 84 24

GA: Looks mildly SOB, pursed-lip breathing

HEENT: Pharynx is clear. No abnormal cervical or supraclavicular adenopathy.

Chest: Prolonged expiratory phase. Chest with increased AP diameter. NL respiratory excursion. Normal tactile fremitus, percussion, and auscultation.

CV: S1, S2 WNL; no murmur, rub, or gallop. No JVD. PMI not displaced.

Ext: No cyanosis or edema. + Clubbing.

SAMPLE PATIENT NOTE

Data Interpretation: *Based on what you have learned from the history and physical examination,* list up to 3 diagnoses that might explain this patient's complaint(s). List your diagnoses from most to least likely. For some cases, fewer than 3 diagnoses will be appropriate. Then, enter the positive or negative findings from the history and the physical examination (if present) that support each diagnosis. Lastly, list initial *diagnostic* studies (if any) you would order for this patient (e.g., restricted physical exam maneuvers, laboratory tests, imaging, ECG, etc.).

Diagnosis #1: Emphysema

Differential diagnosis and diagnostic reasoning

History Finding(s)	**Physical Exam Finding(s)**
DOE	Increased RR
50 pk-yr smoking history	Pursed-lip breathing
Decreased exercise capacity	Prolonged expiratory phase
	Increased AP diameter of chest
	+ clubbing

Diagnosis #2: Tuberculosis

Differential diagnosis and diagnostic reasoning

History Finding(s)	**Physical Exam Finding(s)**
Productive cough, weight loss	

Diagnosis #3: Lung cancer

Differential diagnosis and diagnostic reasoning

History Finding(s)	**Physical Exam Finding(s)**
50 pk-yr smoking hx	
Hemoptysis	
Weight loss	

Diagnostic Study/Studies

CBC

Pulmonary function test

PPD

CT chest

CASE DISCUSSION

Notes about the History-Taking

In this case it is important to get the amount of cigarettes smoked. Find out when he started smoking as well as the course and duration of tobacco use. Ask if the patient ever got treatment and was able to stop. Maximizing information from past failures and successes is key. Asking about complications of tobacco use such as heart disease, lung disease, and symptoms of cancer would be appropriate.

Notes about the Physical Exam

This case requires a complete chest exam as well as some of the cardiovascular exam. Focusing the most attention on the lungs is based on his history of sputum and dyspnea.

Comments about the Patient Note

In this case the smoking history and related symptoms are the HPI. There is no need to mention it again in the social history. It is important to note that although your SPs will not have any "real" acute findings, you may have patients that do have symptoms of chronic illnesses. It would not be unusual to have an SP with changes in the chest wall (e.g., increased chest AP diameter) and possibly signs of clubbing. Don't be surprised to find real physical findings as well as simulated.

Emphysema and chronic obstructive pulmonary disease would also be accepted as correct diagnoses. One pack-year (pk-yr) is defined as smoking one package of cigarettes per day for one year. Screening recommendations call for low-dose chest CT scan in heavy smokers (>30 pack-years) between the ages of 55 and 80. So a CT scan would be warranted in this case even if you weren't concerned about active lung disease.

Case 20: **Bizarre Behavior**

BEFORE ENTERING THE ROOM

Clinical Reasoning: Altered mental status indicates that you will need to complete a neuro exam and a psychiatric exam as well. When you enter the room this patient will be wearing street clothes, so no physical exam will be possible. Do not give the drape to a standardized patient wearing street clothes. You still should do a complete mini mental status exam.

Mental status changes can be caused by psychiatric illness as well as causes that are considered more organic, such as recreational drug use and encephalitis.

The psychiatric exam consists of the following:
- General appearance
- Orientation to person, place, and time
- Speech
- Recent and remote memory

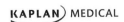

- Attention and concentration
- Mood and affect
- Thought process
- Hallucinations, delusions, or paranoia
- Suicidal/homicidal ideations
- Insight

General appearance is no different from any other case. Simply describe how the patient looks, any poor hygiene, disorganized appearance, and anything out of the ordinary.

A large part of the psychiatric exam is simply the Mini Mental Status exam. In addition to Mini Mental Status, you will need to comment on the patient's speech, mood, and affect, and the presence or absence of hallucinations and/or delusions. Finally, no psychiatric chart is complete without commenting on suicidal ideations.

Speech can be described as normal, pressured, or rapid. Feel free to comment on the volume, rate, tone, and accent, and any stuttering or idiosyncratic features.

Mood is what the patient says in response to questioning about his mood.

Affect is the emotional state that you (as the physician) observe: euthymic, neutral, euphoric, dysphoric, flat, and blunted are all psychological terms. Simply describe, in your own terms, what you see.

Thought process is the organization of the patient's thought process: logical, loose associations, flight of ideas, tangential, and circumstantial are all common descriptors.

Hallucinations

Doctor: "Sometimes people see or hear things that are not really there. Does this ever happen to you?"

Delusions

Doctor: "Do people ever tell you that you have very unusual ideas about yourself or the world?"

Insight is what the patient thinks he needs in terms of treatment.

Doctor: "What do you think about your symptoms (illness)?"

FROM THE STANDARDIZED PATIENT

History

HPI: Mr. Lee is brought to you by the police. Of course, the police have left before you arrive and are unavailable for interview. Mr. Lee is fully dressed, so you know a physical exam involving heart, lungs, and abdomen will not be needed on this case. When you enter the room he is standing, staring at the wall. His clothes are torn and dirty. It looks like he hasn't showered in a week. He appears to be staring intently at a small spot on the wall.

When you call his name he startles and turns to stare at you. To your surprise, he answers questions quite bluntly and efficiently. He tells you he is not sure why he was brought to the doctor. He states that he "on a mission" to stop the university from making any additional mistakes and thereby "save the solar system." He tells you he is a college student in astrophysics at the university. Or rather, he *was* a student until he was expelled for his thesis idea that no one else could understand. He states that he made such a breakthrough while in communication with Alpha Centaurians. He has felt this way for several months. Prior to this he was not so sure about the alien communication, but now he has proof. He tells you that at one time he fit into the establishment and got a full-ride scholarship to the university right out of high school. But over the past two years, as he concentrated on his work to the exclusion of all social contact, he made this discovery. Nothing has made the voices better or worse. He has felt sad, hopeless, or guilty at times. He is somewhat angry about being forced out his apartment and living on the street.

He denies currently using recreational drugs. He smoked marijuana a few times in high school but didn't like losing control. For this reason he rarely drinks alcohol. He also tells you that one of the reasons he doesn't go to parties at school is that he is sure the government would know if he drank illegally. He states he has no allergies. He takes no medications because there "may be a government plot preventing me from saving the solar system."

He was hospitalized once for 3 days last month when he was found talking to himself in the park. The hospital released him with a bottle of pills, which he discarded to prevent government eavesdropping. No trauma. No surgery. No history of high blood sugar or high blood pressure.

He has not been sleeping more than an hour or two a night. He has lost 20 to 30 lb.

Family Hx: There is no family history of psychiatric disease. His father died last year at age 72.

Social Hx: He is not sexually active. He has no family. He does not smoke or use alcohol.

Physical Exam

Mr. Lee is oriented to person, place, and time. He seems intelligent. He frequently uses novel new words and has to explain their meaning. His recent and delayed memory are intact. He will not spell the word *world* backwards to test attention and concentration; he feels that is beneath someone of his stature. He states that he feels elated and honored to be the contact person for the aliens. He looks agitated. He does not feel he needs the attention of a physician because nothing is wrong. His work must not be interrupted. He has no plans to harm himself or anyone else.

In this case you have only general appearance, vital signs, and mental status exam.

THE CLOSING

Doctor: "Mr. Lee, thank you for speaking with me. Thank you for telling me about the voices and the communications you have been receiving. I want to get a blood test to check your sugar and look for any chemical imbalance that could be causing your symptoms."

CHALLENGING QUESTIONS

Mr. Lee: "I don't want any tests. I don't want you to inject me with any monitoring devices."

Doctor: "I'm here to help and would never do anything to harm you. I'll have the counselor come and speak to you now. Do you have any questions?"

SAMPLE PATIENT NOTE

History: Describe the history you just obtained from this patient. Include only information (pertinent positives and negatives) relevant to this patient's problem(s).

CC: *Brought in by police for bizarre behavior.*

HPI: *20 y/o male brought in by police. Pt is hearing voices. Has plan to save solar system. Recently lost his housing. Is a former university student who states he is in communication with aliens. Expresses paranoia about possible government eavesdropping.*

              Symptoms have been continuous for at least 3 months. Nothing has made it better, including a brief hospitalization for similar symptoms last month. Was given medication which he didn't take secondary to paranoid delusions. Not sleeping (1–2 hours/day), 20-lb weight loss. Pt states feels sad and hopeless at times, feels angry over loss of housing at other times. No previous psychotic episodes. Rare current alcohol or recreational drug use, but smoked marijuana a few times in high school.

PMH: *NKMA, noncompliant with any medication*

              Denies trauma, DM, HTN, or surgery.

FH: *No hx of psychiatric illness. Father died last year at age 72.*

SAMPLE PATIENT NOTE

Physical Examination: Describe any positive and negative findings relevant to this patient's problem(s). Be careful to include *only* those parts of examination you performed in *this* encounter.

GA: *Pt is dirty and staring at wall*

VS: *37.2 140/80 90 16*

Psychiatric
history: *Pt is alert and oriented to person, place, and time*

              Speech is rapid and pressured

              Recent and remote memory intact

              Not cooperative to check attention and concentration

              Mood: Expansive, elated

              Affect: Agitated, jittery

              Thought process: Delusional

              + Psychosis, hearing voices of the "aliens"

              Denies suicidal or homicidal intent

SAMPLE PATIENT NOTE

Data Interpretation: *Based on what you have learned from the history and physical examination,* list up to 3 diagnoses that might explain this patient's complaint(s). List your diagnoses from most to least likely. For some cases, fewer than 3 diagnoses will be appropriate. Then, enter the positive or negative findings from the history and the physical examination (if present) that support each diagnosis. Lastly, list initial *diagnostic* studies (if any) you would order for this patient (e.g., restricted physical exam maneuvers, laboratory tests, imaging, ECG, etc.).

Diagnosis #1: Schizophrenia/acute psychosis

Differential diagnosis and diagnostic reasoning

History Finding(s)	Physical Exam Finding(s)
Hearing voices	*Delusional thought process*
Decreased level of functioning	*Oriented with intact memory*
	Out of touch with reality, paranoid delusions

Diagnosis #2: Bipolar with manic episode

Differential diagnosis and diagnostic reasoning

History Finding(s)	Physical Exam Finding(s)
Hearing voices	*Poor concentration*
Not sleeping	*Rapid, pressured speech*
Elated mood	*Delusional thoughts of grandeur*

Diagnosis #3:

Differential diagnosis and diagnostic reasoning

History Finding(s)	Physical Exam Finding(s)

Diagnostic Study/Studies

Physical exam

Drug screen

EtOH

CASE DISCUSSION

Notes about the History-Taking

This patient is blatantly psychotic and is very verbal about what he experiencing. Many patients with schizophrenia have much less speech. The USMLE, however, will not give you a patient with catatonia (there would be no way to test your interpersonal skills and English proficiency).

Many patients are reticent to speak about the voices, and it may take a few minutes for you to realize that the patient is having auditory hallucinations, tangential thinking, loose associations, or bizarre thoughts.

A good way to ask about psychosis if it is:

> **Doctor:** "Sometimes when people are under a lot of stress, they hear or see things that other people do not. Has this ever happened to you?"

Comments about the Patient Note

Always read the Doorway Information carefully, as it will say what the tasks are and if a note and physical are wanted. This patient is wearing street clothes and you will need to include a physical exam in the workup. This is because a patient who is to be examined must first change into a gown.

Write the psychiatric exam in the Physical Exam section of the note.

Case 21: **Diarrhea**

DOORWAY INFORMATION

Opening Scenario

Larry Todd is a 55 y/o man with diarrhea.

Vital Signs

1. Temp: 38.0°C (100.4°F)
2. BP: 120/80 mm Hg
3. HR: 70/min
4. RR: 20/min

Examinee Tasks

1. Obtain a focused history.
2. Perform a relevant physical examination. Do not perform rectal, pelvic, genitourinary, inguinal hernia, female breast, or corneal reflex examinations.
3. Discuss your initial diagnostic impression and your workup plan with the patient.
4. After leaving the room, complete your patient note on the given form.

BEFORE ENTERING THE ROOM

Patients have variable definitions of what constitutes diarrhea. Establish if the patient means watery stools or soft stools, and quantify the number of trips to the bathroom each day. Diarrhea can be caused by infectious agents, so travel history and sick contacts are important. Some foods may cause diarrhea in those who are lactose or fructose intolerant. Medications or inflammatory bowel disease may be the cause. Irritable bowel is a common problem.

From the doorway you can anticipate the need to assess the SP's hydration status and to put infection high on your differential given the patient's low-grade fever. This will also make common problems like irritable bowel and lactose intolerance less likely.

FROM THE STANDARDIZED PATIENT

History

HPI: The patient, Larry Todd, states that his diarrhea started abruptly as brown, watery stool multiple times a day 9 months ago. He had fever, cramps, and vomiting. Mr. Todd had just come back from a camping and hunting trip in the western United States when the symptoms started. After 4–5 days his symptoms started to improve, but now off and on he has all-over abdominal cramping with loose stools 2–3 times per day. Cramps are intense but brief.

The patient has had some weeks where he experiences bloating, some greasy stools, and nausea. The vomiting has stopped. He has not noticed any fever or observed vomit or blood in the stool (no stool that is red or black). He has had a 10-pound unintentional weight loss in the last 3–4 months. He feels less energetic and has a lot of belching. There doesn't seem to be a connection to any particular foods, including dairy.

No one else has had diarrhea. His hunting buddies who went on the trip with him did not get sick.

Patient denies alcohol. He lives with his current girlfriend, has been divorced for 5 years. He has 2 adult children. He is sexually active with his girlfriend and occasionally with men. He doesn't use condoms with his girlfriend but he "almost always" uses them when he has sex with men. He does not identify as either homosexual or bisexual.

PMH: He was hospitalized for gallbladder removal 5 years ago.

Medications: None

Family Hx: One sibling with ulcerative colitis.

Social Hx: He states that he enjoys smoking a good cigar when he can get one. He lives in Washington, D.C., most of the year.

Physical Exam

Patient does not appear to be in acute distress. He has no jaundice. His mucous membranes appear moist. His lungs are clear to auscultation bilaterally. The heart sounds are normal. On inspection of the abdomen, you see no surgical scars. The bowel sounds are hyperactive. The liver and spleen are not enlarged. There is diffuse abdominal tenderness without any rebound in all 4 quadrants. He is hyperresonant in all 4 quadrants.

THE CLOSING

During your closing you can explain what the most likely diagnoses are, what tests will help figure out the case, and suggest that the patient get tested for HIV.

> **Doctor:** "Mr. Todd, you've told me that you've lost some weight, and here we found you to have a bit of a fever. On your exam, I find some tenderness in the belly, which may be from an infection you picked up while camping. I will need to take a stool sample to check for infection. I also strongly recommend an HIV test, since you have had some unprotected sexual encounters."

CHALLENGING QUESTIONS

> **Mr. Todd:** "I'm not gay. Are you saying that you think I have AIDS?"
>
> **Doctor:** "Anyone who has unprotected sex is at risk for HIV, and the greater the number of sexual partners, the greater the risk. Those with HIV are at increased risk for certain types of infectious causes of diarrhea."

SAMPLE PATIENT NOTE

History: Describe the history you just obtained from this patient. Include only information (pertinent positives and negatives) relevant to this patient's problem(s).

CC: 55-y/o man with 9 months of intermittent crampy diarrhea. Denies blood in stool.

HPI: Started suddenly after camping trip. No sick contacts. 2–3 BMs a day.

           No previous episodes. Reports belching, weight loss, and reduced energy. Has multiple sexual partners, MSM unsafe sex, has never had HIV test. Family history of inflammatory bowel disease.

PMH: Gallbladder removal

           No medications, NKDA

SH: Smokes cigars, no EtOH

SAMPLE PATIENT NOTE

Physical Examination: Describe any positive and negative findings relevant to this patient's problem(s). Be careful to include *only* those parts of examination you performed in *this* encounter.

VS: T 38.0, BP 120/80, HR 70, RR 20

GA: NAD

HEENT: Mucous membranes moist

Chest: Lungs clear to A

CV: Heart regular, no MRG

Abd: Appears normal. BS++, hyperresonant to percussion all 4 quadrants. Diffuse tenderness all 4 quadrants. No rebound. No hepatosplenomegaly.

SAMPLE PATIENT NOTE

Data Interpretation: *Based on what you have learned from the history and physical examination*, list up to 3 diagnoses that might explain this patient's complaint(s). List your diagnoses from most to least likely. For some cases, fewer than 3 diagnoses will be appropriate. Then, enter the positive or negative findings from the history and the physical examination (if present) that support each diagnosis. Lastly, list initial *diagnostic* studies (if any) you would order for this patient (e.g., restricted physical exam maneuvers, laboratory tests, imaging, ECG, etc.).

Diagnosis #1: Giardiasis

Differential diagnosis and diagnostic reasoning

History Finding(s)	Physical Exam Finding(s)
9 months diarrhea with cramps	Fever
Occurred after camping trip	Diffuse abdominal tenderness
Weight loss, MSM	
No prior episodes	

Diagnosis #2: Cryptosporidium

Differential diagnosis and diagnostic reasoning

History Finding(s)	Physical Exam Finding(s)
9 months diarrhea with cramps	Fever
Weight loss	Diffuse abdominal tenderness

Diagnosis #3: Crohn disease

Differential diagnosis and diagnostic reasoning

History Finding(s)	Physical Exam Finding(s)
Chronic diarrhea	Fever
Weight loss	Diffuse abdominal tenderness
Family hx IBD	

Diagnostic Study/Studies

Stool for ova and parasites

Stool for fecal leukocytes

CBC, electrolytes, HIV test, CD4 count

Stool for enteric pathogens

Colonoscopy (if other tests for infection are negative)

CASE DISCUSSION

Notes about the History-Taking

Patients may have a sexual identity that does not conform to our preconceived notions based on their sexual behavior. Be careful not to make assumptions about patients' sexuality. Ask questions in a respectful and non-judgmental manner.

Comments about the Patient Note

There are many possible causes of infectious diarrhea that are more frequently found in immunocompromised hosts. You should choose the more common ones based as the patient's risk factors. In addition to cryptosporidium, amebiasis would be an acceptable diagnosis to include, especially given the preceding camping trip.

Case 22: **Chest Pain**

BEFORE ENTERING THE ROOM

Clinical Reasoning: The chest pain differential diagnosis is broad. In this age group with essentially normal vital signs, diagnosis that presents immediate life and limb threats such as any form of myocardial ischemia, aortic dissection, pulmonary embolism, pneumothorax, or Boerhaave syndrome already seems unlikely.

FROM THE STANDARDIZED PATIENT

History

HPI: Ms. Grenelli states she has had a burning feeling in her chest off and on for the past 2 years. She states that the pain is in the center of chest, underneath the breastbone, and sometimes goes from the top of her stomach.

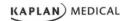

(She points to her epigastric region during the interview when you ask her to show you where it hurts.) The pain moves up to the throat frequently. It does not go to her neck, back, jaw, or arms.

Pain episodes can last anywhere from 15 minutes to several hours and are sometimes relieved with a calcium carbonate tablet. They occur about 3–5 times a week. She notices the problem more after a big meal, when she lies down, and when she bends over to pick up something from the floor.

The pain does not seem to change when she goes for a brisk walk, climbs stairs, or otherwise exerts herself. There is no shortness of breath or sweating. There is no vomiting or diarrhea, and no blood in the stool. There is sometimes nausea and a sour taste when she has reflux of food. She never coughs or chokes. She denies any change in weight and reports that she is 20 pounds overweight since the birth of her second child 2.5 years ago. Previously Ms. Grenelli had heartburn only with pregnancy. Her last period was 2 weeks ago and normal.

She has 2 children, ages 2 and 5. Both were normal deliveries. She has had no surgery, and she does not have diabetes, hypertension, or breathing difficulties.

Social Hx: Ms. Grenelli lives with her husband and 2 children, works as an administrative assistant. She denies the use of recreational drugs. She has an occasional alcoholic beverage and has smoked 1 pack of cigarettes a day for the past 10 years.

Physical Exam

On physical exam, skin and sclera are not jaundiced. Lungs are clear to auscultation anterior and posterior. Heart sounds are normal, without rub, murmur, or gallop. Ms. Grenelli's abdomen appears normal, and bowel sounds are normative. Percussion in each of the 4 quadrants is normal. There is no enlargement of the liver or spleen. There is epigastric tenderness and pressure felt with pressure applied on epigastrium; elsewhere the abdomen is nontender. There is no rebound or Murphy's sign.

THE CLOSING

> **Doctor:** "For the past 2 years you have had a burning, heartburn-like feeling in the chest like you did when you were pregnant. It is worse lying down and sometimes better when you take an antacid." (*Pause for patient to respond.*)

> "On your exam you have a little tenderness in your belly below your chest. I think what you have is most likely heartburn, also known as reflux or GERD. In other words, your symptoms may be due to acid from the stomach moving up into the esophagus, or food tube. It's also possible that the weight gain you experienced with your pregnancy could have caused something called a hiatal hernia, where the stomach sometimes moves up into the chest, which can be very uncomfortable. All of these symptoms might get a lot better if you lose some of the extra weight and stop smoking. We will also check whether you have an infection in your stomach that is causing an ulcer."

CHALLENGING QUESTIONS

> **Ms. Grenelli:** "Can't you just give me a prescription for the 'purple pill' I see advertised on TV?"

> **Doctor:** "A medication like that might help manage your symptoms. But before we try it, we should make sure we know what is causing your symptoms and help you to make some changes that can more permanently control the problem."

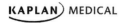

SAMPLE PATIENT NOTE

History: Describe the history you just obtained from this patient. Include only information (pertinent positives and negatives) relevant to this patient's problem(s).

30 y/o female

CC:	*2 yrs burning substernal chest pain, can radiate to throat and epigastrium*
HPI:	*Feels "burning," lasts 15 min. to hours, nonexertional. Happens several times per week. Feels like the same heartburn she had when she was 3rd trimester pregnant.*
	20-lb weight gain since birth of last child but no recent change in weight.
	Worse with large meal, lying down, or bending over. Better with taking calcium carbonate tabs.
	No SOB, vomiting, radiation to back, blood in stool
	+ sour taste of food reflux, with occasional nausea
PMH:	*G2P2, LMP 2 weeks ago; states not pregnant*
	Antacids, no other meds
	No surgery, DM, HTN
SH:	*Lives with husband and 2 children. No recreational drugs. Occasional alcoholic beverage. Currently smokes 1 pk/day (10 pk-yr total).*

SAMPLE PATIENT NOTE

Physical Examination: Describe any positive and negative findings relevant to this patient's problem(s). Be careful to include *only* those parts of examination you performed in *this* encounter.

VS:	*T 37.0, BP 122/84, HR 72, RR 16*
GA:	*Alert, NAD*
HEENT:	*Normal, no jaundice*
Chest:	*Lungs clear to A, heart S1, S2, no RMG*
Abd:	*Appears normal, BS+. No hepatosplenomegaly or rebound. Mild epigastric tenderness. Percussion NL all 4 Q's. Neg Murphy's.*

SAMPLE PATIENT NOTE

Data Interpretation: *Based on what you have learned from the history and physical examination,* list up to 3 diagnoses that might explain this patient's complaint(s). List your diagnoses from most to least likely. For some cases, fewer than 3 diagnoses will be appropriate. Then, enter the positive or negative findings from the history and the physical examination (if present) that support each diagnosis. Lastly, list initial *diagnostic* studies (if any) you would order for this patient (e.g., restricted physical exam maneuvers, laboratory tests, imaging, ECG, etc.)

Diagnosis #1: Gastroesophageal reflux disease

Differential diagnosis and diagnostic reasoning

History Finding(s)	**Physical Exam Finding(s)**
15 min to hours-long episodes of chest discomfort	No jaundice
	Normal vital signs
Nonexertional	
Better with antacids	
Worse with large meal and lying flat	
No vomiting or blood in stool	
Overweight but no recent change in weight	

Diagnosis #2: Hiatal hernia

Differential diagnosis and diagnostic reasoning

History Finding(s)	**Physical Exam Finding(s)**
Chest pain after large meals and when lying down	Mild epigastric tenderness and pressure when epigastrium palpated

Diagnosis #3: Gastritis/peptic ulcer disease

Differential diagnosis and diagnostic reasoning

History Finding(s)	**Physical Exam Finding(s)**
Pain after eating large meal	Tender epigastrium
Better with antacids	

Diagnostic Study/Studies

Rectal exam and stool for occult blood

Esophagogastroduodenoscopy

CBC, amylase, lipase

T. bili, alk phos, ALT, AST

CASE DISCUSSION

Notes about the History-Taking

The fact that this patient's pain started 2 years ago, is not exertional, and can last several hours makes a diagnosis of chest pain that causes immediate loss of life unlikely. Finding out the specific factors that improve or worsen these chronic symptoms will narrow down the possibilities.

Notes about the Physical Exam

The physical exam focuses on the abdominal exam in this case. With the current differential it is not as helpful as the history.

Case 23: **Syncope**

BEFORE ENTERING THE ROOM

Clinical Reasoning: "Collapsed" is one of those lay terms that has no specific meaning but invokes someone who may have fallen, may have fainted, or remains unconscious. Immediately think of a differential diagnosis of syncope at the doorway. The two common and less worrisome causes of syncope are orthostatic hypotension and vasovagal syncope. For more serious reasons for syncope, consider neurogenic and cardiogenic causes. Neurogenic causes include seizure and, more rarely, subarachnoid hemorrhage. Cardiogenic causes include arrhythmia, ischemia, and structural abnormalities. Saddle pulmonary embolism or significant hemorrhage can also cause syncope, but patients are obviously acutely ill upon regaining consciousness.

FROM THE STANDARDIZED PATIENT

History

HPI: Mr. Spade says he doesn't remember what happened. The last thing he remembers is walking from the parking lot to keep a dentist appointment; then there were a lot of people standing around him. He had no warning signs and doesn't remember feeling faint. He is not sure how long he was unconscious but estimates it couldn't have been more than a few minutes. Mr. Spade is very embarrassed that he "wet his pants." The only thing that hurts after his fall is his tongue. He isn't sure if he hit his head, but his head doesn't hurt now. He supposes he fainted, which has not happened since he was best man at a wedding at age 20. Someone in the parking lot called an ambulance, and by the time it came, he was feeling much better and could talk to the EMS workers.

He says he just has not felt well the last 4 months. He has had a diffuse, mild headache (2/10, barely noticeable at times) that is worse in the mornings, and also his family tells him he has been forgetful lately. He admits to being distracted by problems at work and has not been sleeping very well. He has not had any chest pain, shortness of breath, or palpitations. This has never happened before. Mr. Spade usually drinks 2 martinis a day, but he has tried to cut down to one martini a day since he wants to lose weight. He doesn't get annoyed talking about his drinking but does feel like 2 drinks every day is probably too much. On weekends he often has a drink with brunch. His last drink was 2 days ago. He has never had a seizure or trauma. No one in his family has had a seizure. He had a brother who died suddenly at age 49, something to do with his heart.

PMH: Mr. Spade takes no medicine and has no allergies. He has had no surgeries. He does not have a history of diabetes, hypertension, or high cholesterol.

Social Hx: Mr. Spade lives in the suburbs, commutes to work on the train each day, and works as a systems analyst. He does not smoke or use recreational drugs. He is on no special diet.

Physical Exam

When you enter, Mr. Spade is resting comfortably, lying down. He sits up and appears without distress except for his sore tongue.

His head is without injury (except for a little blood on the tip of his tongue). His pupils are equal, round, and reactive to light. His extraocular movements are normal. Pharynx is clear. Upon your request his tongue protrudes straight out. There is no facial asymmetry. His lungs are clear to auscultation. There is no tenderness to palpation to the neck, chest wall, abdomen, or extremities.

His heart is RRR, normal S1 and S2 without any murmurs, heaves, or gallops.

Mr. Spade is alert and oriented to person, place, and time. He moves all 4 extremities equally, and finger-to-nose exam is normal, no asterixis. Cranial nerves are all intact. Motor is 5/5 upper and lower extremities. He can spell "world" backwards and remembers 3 objects.

THE CLOSING

Doctor: "You passed out and don't really remember what happened. I see that you bit your tongue when you fainted in the parking lot. The most likely explanation is that you had a seizure today. It's possible that because you usually have alcohol every day but have skipped a few days that your body is withdrawing from the alcohol. But we also need to check and make sure that your heart is okay. We're going to do some blood tests, check a cardiogram. In addition, we need to do a CT scan of your brain to make sure that there was no damage when you fell."

CHALLENGING QUESTIONS

Mr. Spade: "I feel much better. Can I go home now?"

Doctor: "While it is not certain that what happened was very serious, it is likely enough that you will need to stay in the hospital. We will need to watch your heart rate, blood pressure, and temperature closely to see if you are withdrawing from alcohol. That is a potentially dangerous condition."

SAMPLE PATIENT NOTE

History: Describe the history you just obtained from this patient. Include only information (pertinent positives and negatives) relevant to this patient's problem(s).

CC: Pt had sudden LOC in parking lot.

HPI: Pt was walking in parking lot when he had an unwitnessed syncope. Appears to have bit tongue, and was incontinent of urine. 4 mo Hx of 2/10 headache, mild constant diffuse, worse in mornings. Not sleeping well and distracted by problems at work. Family telling him he's been forgetful lately. Denies CP, SOB, palpitations. EtOH: Usually 2 drinks/day but trying to cut down; last drink 2 days ago. CAGE 2–3 out of 4. No history of seizure. Fainted once at wedding 30+ years ago is only prior episode.

        Family history of early sudden death in brother.

        No medications. NKDA.

PMH: No hospitalizations, surgery, or trauma.

SH: No recreational drug use.

SAMPLE PATIENT NOTE

Physical Examination: Describe any positive and negative findings relevant to this patient's problem(s). Be careful to include *only* those parts of examination you performed in *this* encounter.

VS: T 37.2, BP 150/890, HR 95, RR 16

GA: Pt sitting up with eyes open and NAD.

HEENT: Bite mark on tongue. No tenderness to head otherwise.

Neck: Nontender

Chest: No deformity or tenderness. Lungs clear to A. Heart RRR; NL S1, S2; no murmurs.

Neuro: A + O x 3. PERRL EOMI. No facial asymmetry. Cranial nerves intact. Motor 5/5 all 4 extremities.

        Finger-to-nose intact. Remembers 3 objects. Can spell "world" backward.

SAMPLE PATIENT NOTE

Data Interpretation: *Based on what you have learned from the history and physical examination*, list up to 3 diagnoses that might explain this patient's complaint(s). List your diagnoses from most to least likely. For some cases, fewer than 3 diagnoses will be appropriate. Then, enter the positive or negative findings from the history and the physical examination (if present) that support each diagnosis. Lastly, list initial *diagnostic* studies (if any) you would order for this patient (e.g., restricted physical exam maneuvers, laboratory tests, imaging, ECG, etc.).

Diagnosis #1: Seizure from alcohol withdrawal

Differential diagnosis and diagnostic reasoning

History Finding(s)	Physical Exam Finding(s)
Sudden loss of consciousness	Slight elevation of HR, BP, temp
Incontinent of urine	Bite mark on tongue
Bit tongue	
No alcohol for 2 days after years of daily drinking	

Diagnosis #2: Arrhythmia

Differential diagnosis and diagnostic reasoning

History Finding(s)	Physical Exam Finding(s)
Sudden LOC	No motor weakness or other neurological deficits
Family history sudden death	Mental status normal

Diagnosis #3:

Differential diagnosis and diagnostic reasoning

History Finding(s)	Physical Exam Finding(s)

Diagnostic Study/Studies

CT head

Electrolytes, BUN, Cr, glucose, EtOH

ECG

EEG

CASE DISCUSSION

Comments about the Patient Note

The physical examination includes cardiac exam and neuro exam assessing the mental status, both formally and by observation. The patient doesn't seem postictal but—as is often the case with an unwitnessed syncope that the patient doesn't remember—there will be some holes in the history.

| SECTION 3 |

Appendixes

Appendix A: **Common Abbreviations for the Patient Note**

The following list provided by the USMLE demonstrates the types of abbreviations that are commonly used on the Patient Note of the Step 2 CS exam. Use abbreviations sparingly. For clarity, it is always better to spell out the full form of the acronym or abbreviation.

Units of Measure

C	Celsius
cm	Centimeter
F	Fahrenheit
hr	Hour
kg	Kilogram
lbs	Pounds
mcg	Microgram
mg	Milligram
min	Minute
oz	Ounces

Vital Signs

BP	Blood pressure
HR	Heart rate
R	Respirations
T	Temperature

Routes of Drug Administration

IM	Intramuscularly
IV	Intravenously
po	Orally

Medical Abbreviations

ø	Without or no
+ or pos	Positive
– or neg	Negative
Abd	Abdomen
AIDS	Acquired Immune Deficiency Syndrome
AP	Anteroposterior

CABG	Coronary artery bypass grafting
CBC	Complete blood count
CHF	Congestive heart failure
COPD	Chronic obstructive pulmonary disease
CPR	Cardiopulmonary resuscitation
CT	Computed tomography
CVA	Cerebrovascular accident
CVP	Central venous pressure
CXR	Chest x-ray
DM	Diabetes mellitus
DTR	Deep tendon reflexes
ECG or EKG	Electrocardiogram
ED	Emergency department
EMT	Emergency medical technician
ENT	Ears, nose, and throat
EOM	Extraocular muscles
EtOH	Alcohol
Ext	Extremities
f or ♀	Female
FH or FHx	Family history
GI	Gastrointestinal
GU	Genitourinary
h/o	History of
HEENT	Head, eyes, ears, nose, and throat
HIV	Human immunodeficiency virus
HRT	Hormone replacement therapy
HTN	Hypertension
Hx	History
JVD	Jugular venous distention
L	Left
LMP	Last menstrual period
LP	Lumbar puncture
m or ♂	Male
Meds	Medications
MI	Myocardial infarction
MRI	Magnetic resonance imaging
MVA	Motor vehicle accident
Neuro	Neurologic
NIDDM	Non insulin-dependent diabetes mellitus
NKA	No known allergies
NKDA	No known drug allergy
nl	Normal/normal limits
PA	Posteroanterior
PERRLA	Pupils equal, round and reactive to light and accommodation
PMH or PMHx	Past medical history
PT	Prothrombin time
PTT	Partial thromboplastin time

R	Right
RBC	Red blood cells
ROM	Range of motion
SH or SHx	Social history
SOB	Shortness of breath
TIA	Transient ischemic attack
U/A	Urinalysis
URI	Upper respiratory tract infection
WBC	White blood cells
wnl	Within normal limits
yo	Year-old

Appendix B: Communication and Interpersonal Skills (CIS) Behavior List

Functions	Subfunctions
1. Fostering the Relationship	Expressed interest in the patient as a person
	Treated the patient with respect
	Listened and paid attention to the patient
2. Gathering Information	Encouraged the patient to tell his/her story
	Explored the patient's reaction to the illness or problem
3. Providing Information	Provided information related to the working diagnosis
	Provided information on next steps
4a. Making Decisions: Basic	Elicited the patient's perspective on the diagnosis and next steps
	Finalized plans for the next steps
4b. Making Decisions: Advanced	*Sub functions yet to be developed*
5a. Supporting Emotions: Basic	Facilitated the expression of an implied or stated emotion or something important to him/her
5b. Supporting Emotions: Advanced	*Sub functions yet to be developed*
6. Helping Patients with Behavior Change	*Sub functions yet to be developed*

Source: usmle.org

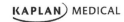

Appendix C: **Differentials and Common Supporting Documentation for Assorted Chief Complaints**

The list that follows is not meant to be exhaustive of all possibilities. It does not limit what should be asked or examined and used as supporting documentation for your diagnosis. Rather, it is meant as a starting point to begin your own thinking.

HEADACHE

Tension

History	Physical
bandlike headache—bilateral	normal vital signs
last for hours	normal neuro exam
recurrent	
constant, not throbbing	
better with massage	

Classic migraine

History	Physical
unilateral or bilateral throbbing	no fever
photophobia, phonophobia	normal neuro exam
nausea	
aura/prodrome	
recurrent	
lasts for hours or days	

Temporal arteritis

History	Physical
age over 50 throbbing one-sided headache low-grade fever or afebrile jaw pain visual changes	tender over temporal artery

Sinusitis

History	Physical
recent upper respiratory infection pain in cheek below eye or "toothache" dull, constant ache, worse leaning over colored nasal discharge and stuffiness	tenderness to palpation of maxillary or frontal sinus inflamed, swollen nasal mucosa

Glaucoma (closed angle)

History	Physical
pain centered over eye first episode	red eye decreased visual acuity dilated pupil

Subdural hematoma

History	Physical
history of trauma on warfarin headache	mental status changes ataxia focal weakness visual changes

Cluster headache

History	Physical
unilateral	lacrimation
sudden and intense	blushing of face
pain behind the eye	
lasts a couple of hours and gone	
recurrent same time of day	

Subarachnoid bleed

History	Physical
headache	mental status changes
syncope	stiff neck
very severe intensity	
first episode	
vomiting	

CHEST PAIN

Acute coronary syndrome

History	Physical
heavy substernal pressure feeling	diaphoretic
shortness of breath	abnormal vital signs
nausea	no high fever
diaphoresis	Levine sign (clenched fist held over chest)
lasts minutes to starting couple hours ago	
risk factors male over age 40 or postmenopausal woman, smoking, family history, diabetes, hypertension, high cholesterol	

Pulmonary embolism

History	Physical
pleuritic chest pain	tachycardia
shortness of breath	tachypnea
unilateral swollen lower leg	no pain to palpation of chest wall
hx of DVT in past	unilateral swollen leg
not on warfarin	

Pneumonia

History	Physical
pleuritic chest pain	fever
cough	dullness to percussion
sputum production	abnormal breath sounds
	increased tactile fremitus

Pneumothorax

History	Physical
pleuritic unilateral chest pain	tachycardia
sudden onset	tachypnea
shortness of breath	decreased unilateral breath sounds
	decreased tactile fremitus

Aortic dissection

History	Physical
ripping chest pain or back pain	blood pressure difference between arms
sudden onset	heart murmur (if aortic insufficiency)
pain radiates to neck or back	pulse differences between sides

Pericarditis

History	Physical
pain better sitting up and leaning forward	cardiac rub
pleuritic	fever
started after viral URI	

Costochondritis

History	Physical
sharp pain hurts with movement and twisting	point tenderness causing the pain

Herpes zoster

History	Physical
unilateral paresthesia of skin unilateral dermatome	unilateral blistering rash on a dermatome fever

Esophageal reflux

History	Physical
heartburn sour taste coming up to mouth pregnant better with antacids pain worse if lies down after eating	no fever no pleuritic pain no abdominal pain

SHORTNESS OF BREATH

Heart failure

History	Physical
dyspnea on exertion pedal edema orthopnea hx of HTN, smoking, coronary disease	rales in lungs gallop heart rhythm (S3, S4) distended neck vein (JVD) distended liver

Chronic obstructive pulmonary disease

History	Physical
dyspnea cough weight loss pursed lip breathing chronic condition, smoking hx	tachypnea increased chest AP diameter clubbing of fingers decreased air entry prolonged expiratory phase

Asthma

History	Physical
recurrent attacks of dyspnea	wheezing
cough	
wheezing	
hx of allergies	
family history of asthma/allergies	

Anemia

History	Physical
fatigue	pallor (conjunctiva, nail beds)
generalized weakness	

Airway obstruction

History	Physical
sudden onset	stridor
change in voice	cyanosis
choked on food or denture	

Myocardial infarction with CHF

History	Physical
substernal chest pain lasting more than 15 min	diaphoresis
dyspnea	(list any abnormal vital signs)
nausea	
hx of smoking, HTN	

Anaphylaxis

History	Physical
acute shortness of breath	hives
wheezing	hypotension
hx of exposure to allergen	tachypnea
	tachycardia

RIGHT UPPER ABDOMINAL PAIN

Biliary colic

History	Physical
RUQ pain—intermittent	no fever
can last several hours	tender right upper quadrant
occurs after fatty meal	
risk factors: female, overweight, pregnant	

Cholecystitis

History	Physical
RUQ pain	fever
radiates to R scapula	+ Murphy's sign
	tender right upper quadrant

Peptic ulcer disease

History	Physical
epigastric RUQ pain	epigastric and RUQ tenderness
taking aspirin or NSAIDs	
blood in stool	
pain may radiate to back	

Pancreatitis

History	Physical
epigastric and RUQ pain	epigastric and RUQ tenderness
pain after eating	
nausea/vomiting	
hx of alcoholism	
hx of gallstone	

Acute hepatitis B

History	Physical
fever	jaundice
jaundice	tender enlarged liver
RUQ pain	– Murphy's sign
hx of unprotected sex, IV drug use	fever

CHRONIC COUGH

Asthma

History	Physical
recurrent attacks of dyspnea	wheezing
cough	
wheezing	
hx of allergies	
family hx of asthma/allergies	

Allergic rhinitis

History	Physical
runny nose	rhinorrhea
itchy watery eyes	watery eyes
recurrent with season	allergic shiners
intermittent hoarse voice/phlegm in throat	cobblestoning in posterior pharynx

Gastroesophageal reflux

History	Physical
heartburn	no fever
sour taste coming up to mouth	no pleuritic pain
pregnant	no abdominal pain
better with antacids	

Chronic obstructive pulmonary disease

History	Physical
dyspnea	tachypnea
cough	increased chest AP diameter
weight loss	clubbing of fingers
pursed lip breathing	decreased air entry
chronic condition, smoking hx	prolonged expiratory phase

Pneumonia

History	Physical
pleuritic chest pain	fever
cough	dullness to percussion
sputum production	abnormal breath sounds
	increased tactile fremitus

ACE inhibitor

History	Physical
taking ACE inhibitor	no fever
dry, nonproductive cough	normal lung exam

Tuberculosis

History	Physical
chronic cough	fever
hemoptysis	lung findings
weight loss	low weight
exposure to TB	
night sweats	

Pulmonary malignancy

History	Physical
hx of smoking	weight loss
cough	wheezing
chest pain	
shortness of breath	
hemoptysis	

ACUTE PELVIC PAIN

Appendicitis

History	Physical
midabdominal pain migrating to RLQ	RLQ tenderness
anorexia	+ obturator sign
nausea/vomiting	+ psoas sign
feverish	fever
acute onset	

Diverticulitis

History	Physical
LLQ pain	fever
fever	LLQ tenderness
diarrhea often	
vomiting	

Pelvic inflammatory disease

History	Physical
fever	fever
lower abdominal pain	lower abdominal tenderness
vaginal discharge	+ pain with cervical motion tenderness
hx of unprotected sex, new sexual partner	shuffling gait

Ectopic pregnancy

History	Physical
lower abdominal pain	lower abdominal tenderness
may radiate to top of shoulder	unilateral adnexal fullness
late period or known pregnant	possible hypotension (if ruptured)

Ovarian torsion

History	Physical
sudden onset	lower abdominal tenderness
unilateral, severe pelvic pain	
nausea and vomiting	
can start with exercise	

BLOOD IN STOOL

Hemorrhoid

History	Physical
bright red blood	no abdominal tenderness
streaks usually on stool or toilet paper	no fever
hx of patient able to palpate hemorrhoid	

Anal fissure

History	Physical
pain with defecation	no fever
bright red blood with straining at stool	no abdominal tenderness

Diverticulosis

History	Physical
abdominal cramps	age > 40
blood mixed with stool	pallor
may be recurrent	

Infectious diarrhea

History	Physical
diarrhea prominent	fever
bloody stool	diffuse abdominal tenderness
vomiting	no rebound
others with same illness	
acute onset	

Inflammatory bowel disease

History	Physical
fever	fever
diarrhea	diffuse abdominal tenderness
chronic onset	
weight loss	
positive family history	

SYNCOPE

Vasovagal

History	Physical
emotional, stressful situation	normal vital signs (when recovered)
quick recovery in minutes	
no seizure activity	
occurred in bathroom	

Arrhythmia

History	Physical
palpitations	abnormal heart rate
chest discomfort	irregular heartbeat
shortness of breath	
medication history	

Orthostatic hypotension

History	Physical
symptoms upon standing, esp. after lying down for a long period of time	tachycardia
medication as cause	hypotension when standing
dehydration	advanced age

Aortic stenosis

History	Physical
shortness of breath	age 60 and up
anginal chest discomfort	narrow pulse pressure
family history of same	displaced PMI
	systolic ejection murmur

Hypertrophic cardiomyopathy

History	Physical
palpitations	crescendo-decrescendo midsystolic heart murmur
dizziness	
shortness of breath	
younger athlete	
family history	
occurs with exercise	

UNILATERAL SWOLLEN LEG

Baker cyst rupture

History	Physical
previous or current arthritis of knee	swelling and fullness behind knee or upper calf
red, swollen, tender calf	

Cellulitis

History	Physical
red, swollen, tender calf	fever
distal break in skin of leg	inguinal adenopathy

Lymphatic obstruction

History	Physical
chronic leg swelling	no fever
chronic skin changes	inguinal adenopathy
not red or tender	lower abdominal mass

Deep vein thrombosis

History	Physical
pain and swelling recently in leg	lower leg red
risk factor for hypercoagulable state (OCPs, ERT, malignancy)	lower leg warm
	lower leg swollen
recent airplane or long bus ride	lower leg tender

BILATERAL SWOLLEN LEGS

Heart failure

History	Physical
dyspnea on exertion	rales in lungs
pedal edema	gallop heart rhythm
orthopnea	distended neck vein
hx of HTN, smoking, coronary disease	distended liver

Nephrotic syndrome

History	Physical
foamy urine	edema bilaterally
weight gain	
edema also around face	
fatigue	

Liver failure

History	Physical
jaundice	jaundice (skin, hard palate, sclera)
fatigue	ascites
right upper quadrant pain	right upper quadrant tenderness
	mental status changes
	edema bilaterally
	asterixis

Obesity/venous insufficiency

History	Physical
pain, swelling in legs	red legs and ankles with darkened skin changes
elevated body mass index	bilateral edema

VOMITING

Note: Be as specific as possible in selecting the diagnosis. For a symptom as general as vomiting it is helpful to think of possible causes based on organ system or other groupings as shown below. For the actual exam, be specific. For example, in the first section below, write "Vomiting from chemotherapy," not "Vomiting from medication."

Medications (chemotherapy, general anesthesia, opioids)

History	Physical
temporal history of medications followed by vomiting	no fever
no blood in emesis	abdomen soft, nontender
vomiting	

Gastroenteritis (rotavirus, norovirus, food poisoning, Campylobacter)

History	Physical
sick contacts or those sharing food also sick	possible fever
abdominal cramps and pain	soft abdomen
diarrhea possible	diffuse abdominal tenderness
vomiting	

Benign paroxysmal positional vertigo (BPPV)

History	Physical
triggered by movement of head	possible nystagmus
vertigo	
vomiting	

Cerebellar (posterior basilar artery) stroke

History	Physical
severe vertigo (may be unable to open eyes)	vertical nystagmus
falling	ataxia
vomiting	dysmetria
	+ Romberg sign

Endocrine and toxins (alcohol, diabetic ketoacidosis)

History	Physical
weakness, fatigue	dry mucous membranes
dehydration	
darkening of skin	
vomiting	